Diet &
Heart Disease

It's Not What You Think...

The book that will change your view of
heart disease and will put good food
back on your table *forever!*

by

STEPHEN BYRNES, ND, RNCP

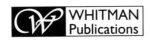

ISBN: 1-885653-14-X

Copyright © 2001 by Wendell W. Whitman Company
302 E. Winona Ave., Warsaw, IN 46580

Cover design by Jason Souther/Rod Weaver.

Webpage: http://www.powerhealth.net

Other titles by Stephen Byrnes:
  Overcoming AIDS with Natural Medicine (1997)
  Digestion Made Simple (2001)

Note to reader: This book is offered for informational purposes only and should not be construed as medical advice. For medical problems, always seek the help of a qualified health professional.

ABOUT THE AUTHOR

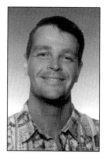 Stephen Byrnes grew up in New York and attended Hunter College in New York City where he received his B.A. in Comparative Religion. After moving to Los Angeles, he completed his M.A. in Humanities at California State University at Dominguez Hills. He then received his Diplomate in Homeobotanical Therapy from the Australasian College of Herbal Studies, a state-licensed college in Lake Oswego, Oregon. In 1998, he earned his Ph.D. in Alternative Medicine with specializations in Clinical Nutrition and Naturopathy from the Canadian Alternative Medicines Research Institute, a government licensed and accredited post-secondary school in Vancouver, British Columbia. Dr. Byrnes is also a Senior Professor of the Institute. Stephen is a board certified Naturopathic Doctor through the American Naturopathic Medical Certification & Accreditation Board (www.anma.com). He is also licensed as a Naturopathic Physician within the state of Idaho, and as a Naturopathic Doctor in Washington, D.C. He also holds registration as a Nutritional Therapist with the International Organization of Nutritional Consultants (http://nutrenet.ionc.com).

Dr. Byrnes has had over 100 articles and papers published in health magazines and professional journals around the world. He also works for a clinic specializing in the holistic treatment of the elderly and the immune-suppressed. He is on the advisory board of the Weston A. Price Foundation and the editorial board of the magazines *WellBeing* (Australia) and *Healthy & Natural* (USA).

With his extensive teaching and writing experience, Dr. Byrnes began the Academy of Natural Therapies, an accredited distance learning institution, to spread the teachings of natural health to all. To learn more about the Academy and its programs, as well as to subscribe to Dr. Byrnes' free bi-monthly ezine, *Health on the Edge*, visit his website at www.PowerHealth.net.

Thanks & Acknowledgements

The author thanks Sally Fallon, MA, for her gracious assistance and patience; the Price-Pottenger Nutrition Foundation for permission to reprint some of Dr. Price's photos; and H. Leon Abrams, Jr., MA, EDS, for stimulating conversations and permission to use his material. Other thanks are due to: Lee Clifford, MS, CCN; Boyd Landry of the Coalition for Natural Health; Wendell Whitman, ND; WellBeing Magazine; and the American Naturopathic Medical Association of Las Vegas, NV. A very special thanks to Danielle Dax for musical inspiration during the preparation of this manuscript.

Table of Contents

NOTE TO THE READER: The information in this book is offered as information only and should not be construed as medical advice. For medical treatment, always seek the help of a qualified medical professional.

Introduction

At the turn of the century, heart disease and atherosclerosis were virtually unheard of. Today, however, they are the Western world's number one killers, with cancer running right behind. As a practitioner who has examined many people, I know that clogged arteries and poor circulation are an unfortunate fact of life for many. While mortality statistics at the turn of the century are not altogether reliable, there is always a consistent figure for deaths from heart attacks or heart disease: between 6-8%. By the 1950s, that number had climbed to 30%. Today, almost 50% of all deaths in the United States and Australia are from cardiovascular disease (CVD) or coronary heart disease (CHD). What went wrong?

As we shall see in this little book, the answers will suprise you. Most of the public (as well as most medical professionals) believe that CVD and CHD are mostly caused by an improper diet and in this they are correct. Where they go wrong, however, is in the elements of that diet. It is very common to hear such nutritional mantras as, "Saturated fat clogs arteries," and "Don't eat too much cholesterol--it's bad for your heart." These assertions are false. Suprised? You should be. The very diet that has been recommended to reduce heart disease by many medical and nutritional practitioners for the past 50 years is the very diet that CAUSES it!

Heart disease is a very complex rubric of different causes with diet being a major, but not the only component. It is hoped that this book will enlighten all who read it. It is hoped that you will avoid heart disease by following the instructions in this volume. In the meantime, take this little "Heart Health Knowledge" quiz to see how much accurate information you hold concerning the heart.

Heart Health Knowldge Quiz

Answer true or false.

___ 1. Saturated fat and cholesterol clog arteries.

___ 2. Vegetarians have lower rates of atherosclerosis and heart disease than non-vegetarians.

___ 3. Eating foods high in cholesterol or saturated fats increases your risk of heart disease.

___ 4. Margarine is better than butter for the heart and circulatory system.

___ 5. Coconut oil is bad for the heart.

___ 6. Using polyunsaturated vegetable oils (corn, safflower, canola, soy, etc) for cooking is better for the heart than butter, cream, lard, or tallow.

___ 7. EKG's are a good way to assess the health of the heart.

___ 8. Angioplasty and bypass operations extend life for heart patients.

___ 9. Most people who die of heart attacks have high cholesterol levels.

___ 10. Reducing your dietary intake of saturated fat and cholesterol is good for you.

All of the above statements are FALSE.
In this book, you'll find out why.

Now its time to test yourself and the health of your heart.

Do you have any of the following?

___ 1. Fingers or toes that often go cold

___ 2. Arms or legs that often "go to sleep"

___ 3. Numbness or heaviness in the arms or legs

___ 4. Cramping in your hand when writing

___ 5. A sharp, diagonal crease in your earlobe

___ 6. Tingling lips or fingers

___ 7. Achy legs after taking a short walk

___ 8. Poor memory

___ 9. Ankles that swell in the later part of the day

___ 10. A whitish ring around the perimeter of your iris

If you answered YES to any of these questions, you could have heart or arterial problems that demand attention. This book will show you how to incorporate natural therapies into your life to reduce and/or eliminate these symptoms. One word of warning, this book is not a substitute for expert help from a qualified health professional. Nor is it designed to diagnose or treat any disease. Do NOT discontinue any medications from your doctor without getting an OK from a qualified health professional.

THE ADVENTURE BEGINS

As we venture into our first chapter together, I ask you to keep an open mind. A lot of what you'll read in this book will directly conflict with what you've heard or read from the health media, your doctor, or establishment dieticians. While it is uncommon for health professionals to deny the Lipid Hypothesis of heart disease, it is certainly not unheard of. From the very beginning, many in the medical field voiced their strenuous objections to the theory that saturated fats and cholesterol caused CVD. The problem is that their views are rarely publicized or ignored. The powerful conglomerate of food processing companies (which make a brisk dollar off of low fat, low cholesterol concoctions of fabricated foods), pharmaceutical companies (which make an even brisker dollar off of cholesterol-lowering drugs), and the establishment, orthodox dietetics associations (which regularly receive monetary "grants" from those corporations), have done a wonderful job of brainwashing the public into dietary practices that have not made a dent in the skyrocketing rates of heart disease, or other chronic diseases such as diabetes and cancer. Believe it. CVD rates have continued to steadily climb in the 50 years that the low saturated fat/cholesterol and high polyunsaturated fat diet has held sway. This has made a lot of money for the beneficiaries of this diet, including funeral homes and coffin makers, but it has not done anything for the general public. Did you know, for example, that low blood cholesterol levels are strongly correlated with high rates of depression, suicide, violent behavior, and cancer? Such is the extent of misinformation fed to the public.

What this book will tell you is how to keep your heart healthy with the use of whole foods and natural substances. It will NOT instruct you in the uses of new fangled, phony foods and dangerous drugs: the children of Modern Technology. So fasten your seatbelts, friends, and get ready to fly. A healthy heart is waiting for you!

CHAPTER ONE

Cause for Concern: The Rise of Cardiovascular Disease

CASE HISTORIES

Phil came to see me on the recommendation of his massage therapist. Standing about 6' 3" and weighing around 325 lbs, Phil had a host of health problems that he knew he had to do something about, but lacked the proper motivation. His massage therapist kept chiding him until he made an appointment with me.

A medical history revealed recurrent gout, adult-onset diabetes, high blood pressure, obesity, and sexual dysfunction. Phil also complained about numbness in his hands and feet. Indeed, his legs from his calves down were discolored, indicating poor circulation. Careful questioning, however, revealed a deep desire to overcome his difficulties. He was, after all, only 48 years old. "I see old Japanese ladies visiting my camp site at the ranch [where he works]. They're in their 70s, riding horses, laughing it up, very active. I'm not even close to 70 and I can't do what they do. I don't want that. I want to be able to jump on a horse for a two hour ride when I'm 70, when I'm 80, and when I'm 90."

Despite his diabetes, Phil consumed a considerable amount of sugar. He loved danishes and pastries. He always had a soft drink with lunch. Until the gout appeared, he wound down the day with a beer and took wine with dinner occasionally. Phil ate a lot of white rice, macaroni salad (made with soybean oil mayonnaise), and an assortment of sweets.

1

My suggestions to him were primarily dietary and, luckily, Phil was willing to take them. Changing food habits is one of the hardest things a nutritionist faces with his clients. Phil also received a vitamin/ mineral formula specifically designed to clear out deposits and plaque from the arteries, as well as various herbal blends to address his blood pressure, gout, diabetes, and poor circulation.

The dietary advice was to avoid large amounts of red meat until the herbs I dispensed could flush out the excessive uric acid from his system. I urged him to eat more fish, properly prepared whole grains, and steamed vegetables, along with moderate amounts of fresh fruit. The main restriction, however, was the one thing Phil enjoyed the most: sugar. I told him in no uncertain terms that refined sugars were the main reason his circulation and health were failing. I gave him some alternatives to sweet foods, as well as an herbal blend to stabilize his blood sugar (to decrease sugar cravings), and sent him on his way.

A month later Phil returned. He was smiling: "If it didn't work, I wouldn't be back here. My legs don't hurt in the morning like they used to and the tingling is gone. My blood pressure has dropped to normal and I've reduced my blood pressure medicine [with his doctor's OK]. My blood sugar has dropped from 300 to 145, so I've cut back on my diabetes medicine. I'm more positive for sure. Oh yeah, I've lost 26 lbs. My energy is incredible—I go hiking now for two and three hours at a time with no problems—I couldn't do that before." I asked Phil about his sexual problem and he wryly grinned at me, "My wife smiles now, too."

In the months that followed, the discoloration on Phil's legs faded and his blood sugar continued to drop. He also lost more weight. Most importantly, he's avoided the sweets and opted for fruits instead, or small amounts of maple syrup or honey.

Dale attended a lecture I gave at a local church on the elements of good nutrition. After the lecture, he made an appointment. Dale, like Phil, was also diabetic, though he was considerably older (70). Dale's main problem was severe edema in his lower legs and very poor circulation. He related to me that earlier in the year he had to go to the hospital because the edema was so bad and his legs ached tremendously after walking just 100 meters. Upon strict orders from his doctor and the hospital dietician, Dale was eating a high complex carbohydrate, low protein, low fat diet. Because he was taking medicine for his blood sugar, Dale ate sweets with impunity. At the time he was very obese and, like Phil, was impotent.

Before he came to see me, Dale had discovered a book by Dr. Robert Atkins, MD, called *Dr. Atkins' New Diet Revolution.* For those of you who are unfamiliar with Atkins' work, he favors a high protein and fat, low carbohydrate diet for weight loss, and a host of diseases, including heart disease. When Dale read the list of health dangers from eating too many carbohydrates, "It was like I was reading my own hospital records!" Dale immediately dropped all grains, sugars, and fruits from his diet and began eating a high meat and saturated fat diet supplemented with ample amounts of fresh vegetables, salads, and nuts. He lost 76 lbs in four months! His blood sugar also dropped, but it was still very high and he responded poorly to the medicines his doctor gave him.

Although Dale knew he had made the right choice by adopting the Atkins' diet plan, he still had problems and came to see me. My intake analysis revealed that Dale's kidneys and pancreas were very weak (I expected as much, however). The edema was incredible, his lower legs and feet were discolored (like Phil's) and when I pressed into his puffy feet, it took a few seconds for the skin to get back to its original state. Because of his health and sexual problems, he was also quite depressed. Dale also had a lingering breathing problem: he would awake every morning with thick mucous deep in his lungs that made it hard to breathe until he coughed it up. At times he would awake at night struggling to breathe due to the mucous blockage.

I placed Dale on the same vitamin/mineral formula as Phil. Additionally, I dispensed diuretic herbs to flush water out from his tissues and to strengthen his kidneys. Other herbs for his blood sugar, circulation, and impotence were also given. Since his diet was working for him, I suggested few changes there, but did point out that certain foods were effective diuretics (asparagus, watermelon, and parsley) and that he should try to add more of those to his meals. I also dispensed some glandular extracts for his pancreas and kidneys, hoping to strengthen them. I instructed Dale to firmly massage the foot reflexes to his kidneys and pancreas twice a day. These two areas were incredibly sensitive, indicating deep tissue weakness.

A month later, Dale happily reported that he was able to walk up to five long blocks before he had to stop to rest. This was a major improvement. His sleep difficulties and breathing problems had dissipated as well. His blood sugar had dropped, but was still elevated. His depression lifted and he lost some weight. Since his edema remained very resistant, however, his weight would sometimes go up due to the extra water weight.

During the months I worked with Dale his energy and circulation continued to improve, but his edema remained very stubborn: he did not respond to either natural or drug remedies (his allopathic doctor, in exasperation, declared Dale a "medical freak"!).

When I asked Dale about his life-style in his earlier days, he said that he followed the standard American diet of refined foods, sweets, sodas, and white grains. He specifically stated that throughout his life, he had used margarine and corn oil instead of butter and other animal fats. Phil had revealed the same thing.

THINGS WEREN'T ALWAYS THIS BAD

As mentioned in the introduction, ◆*heart disease was a rarity in Western countries until the late 1920s* when things definitely started to change for the worse. At the turn of the century, deaths from heart disease were a mere 6% of the total mortality rate. As we shall see in chapter four, the dietary habits of Western peoples at that time were the very habits demonized by modern medicine and nutrition. People ate a lot of saturated fat from various sources including cream and lard.

A number of factors served to increase the rates of heart disease. One of them is the main focus of this book— dietary change. But another, less well-known factor, was the improved sanitation of major cities: as people lived in cleaner environments, rates of infectious disease like tuberculosis and pneumonia, major killers in earlier times, dropped. This "clean-up" occurred primarily with the invention and acceptance of the automobile, which replaced the horse as a means of transport. City streets were often loaded with horse manure. Manure brings flies. Flies bring disease. Coinciding with the decrease in unsanitary wastes was the installation of better plumbing to bring cleaner water to people, and carry dangerous refuse away. Improved housing also did much to reduce the incidence of infectious disease and death. When lots of people are packed closely together in an unsanitary environment, sickness spreads easily and quickly. (It is no coincidence that the Black Plague in Europe originated in the cities.) Obviously, when people live longer they can reach the heart attack age.

TECHNOLOGY'S BLESSING & CURSE

I like to tell audiences I lecture to about a "typical" patient who comes to me for naturopathic counseling. He always begins by saying, "Its just a precaution. I'm actually quite healthy—I have some minor problems, however, that my regular doctor can't seem to help me with, so I thought I'd try this." When I take his medical history, I discover a plethora of problems that would hardly qualify one to be "quite healthy."

This man, we'll call him Joe, had his tonsils removed when he was seven from severe and recurrent throat infections. He also suffered from chronic ear infections as a child, cured by antibiotics. Joe had to get eye glasses the previous year for his ever worsening sight. He has had three root canals, as well as six cavities filled in the last eight years. Joe also suffers from fatigue and bouts of depression—he always attributes these problems to "getting older," and "work-related stress." Joe also tells me of chronic indigestion and gas for which his doctor has prescribed a powerful antacid. Joe has had ulcers in the past as well. About once every two weeks, he needs to take a laxative for his constipation. Joe also reluctantly tells me, with his voice hushed and eyes down, that lately he's been having "sexual problems" and can't seem to perform regularly in the bedroom. He's been thinking of taking that new drug for male impotence (in America), *Viagra*. Lastly, he shows me the eczema on his leg: "I've tried everything for it! It never seems to go away!"

Out of curiosity, I ask Joe about his family. Joe proceeds to tell me of his older sister who died three years ago of breast cancer at the age of 47. His father died of a stroke about a decade ago and his mother was just diagnosed with Alzheimer's disease. Joe's wife gave birth to their two children by Caesarean section and she is slightly obese. She also shares Joe's eczema. Joe's son suffers from asthma, which he's had since he was a child, and attention deficit disorder. Joe assures me that his son is actually "quite smart," but just can't seem to settle down enough to get good grades. His son, now 14, was just fitted for braces. Joe's daughter, a very pretty 9-year old, also wears braces and, like her older brother, has a mouth full of cavities. She also suffers from synovitis, an inflammatory disease of the joints, caused by a chronic streptococcal infection—she is constantly on antibiotics.

No, I am not exaggerating. Many of you reading this might be shocked that you're reading something very similar to your own family history as well. Unfortunately, if we are not such people, we all know others like this. The problem is that, like Joe, we seem to accept these conditions as "normal" and a part of everyday living. We seem to forget that our natural state is one of balance and health—the way our Creator intended.

So Joe, my "typical patient," is most definitely not "quite healthy," as he says. What actually allows him to claim that he is, however, is the very same thing that allows him to turn on the air conditioner, drive to work, send E-mail, and talk to his demented mother long distance—modern technology. Without the tonsillectomy, antibiotics, and eye-glasses, Joe would probably be unable to speak, deaf, and blind (if he was able to survive childhood). Without the dental work, antacids, and laxatives, he'd be a toothless invalid unable to digest his food and a prime candidate for colon cancer. Without a doctor assisting her, Joe's wife would have died during childbirth. Without an inhaler, Joe's son would of died long ago from an asthma attack. Without antibiotics, Joe's daughter would die from a massive bacterial infection. Without expensive orthodontics, Joe's children would have deformed faces from badly-formed teeth.

While technology allows Joe and his family the appearance of health, it does not confer the substance. Technology may be able to get Joe to work across town in ten minutes, but it is not able to cure him of his impotence or other health problems. It did not save his sister from breast cancer. It did not save his father from a stroke, nor his mother from senile dementia. The remedies offered to Joe's children for their health problems are palliative at best, dangerous at worst.

Ironically, and tragically, it is modern technology's tampering with our food supply that has brought many people to their knees. Most individuals do not make the connection between technology and health, but it is there nonetheless. As people gained the benefits of the automobile, the telephone, and the electric light bulb, among many other inventions, we also gained the benefits of convenience foods— frozen dinners, ready-made breads and baked goods, snack foods, and more. No more do we have to milk the cow twice a day for milk, butter, cream, and cheese; now we buy those things in a supermarket. No more do we have to hunt for meat; now we buy it prepackaged. No more do we have to plant grains and vegetables, or pick fruits or nuts; those things are done for us by large farms which practice commercial agriculture.

Modern technological food advances may allow us less time in the kitchen, but we have paid a terrible price for it with our health. Make no mistake about it reader, ◆ *as our food supply has "advanced," so have rates of chronic disease, including heart disease.* We may have processed "cheese foods" that melt easily and work better for cooking, and which stay fresh, unrefrigerated, for several years, but that product is very high in inorganic sodium, aluminum and oxidized cholesterol—all implicated in serious diseases. It contains a fair share of colorings, preservatives, and additives that food scientists don't know too much about in terms of their long term consumption. We may have sugary snack foods that give us a lift when we need some quick energy, but that refined sugar depresses the immune system and contributes to a host of diseases, from diabetes to cancer. We may have crunchy potato or corn chips to eat along with our sandwich, but those chips are coated with refined salt and were cooked in heated vegetable oils which are full of free radicals, potent carcinogens. And on and on it goes.

Worse still, a certain *attitude* goes along with modern technology and its propagators: it's called "pride." This attitude is typical of many in medicine and nutrition today, as well as the other sciences. It is the belief that humans, because of their supposedly advanced knowledge, can do things better than Nature. Not only does mankind have the audacity to *create* an imitation cheese food, it has the gall to assert that *it's better than real cheese!* As another example, food companies scrambled (no pun intended) to create a cholesterol-free "egg" when establishment nutritionists declared real eggs to be unhealthy.

"Egg Beaters™" were introduced to the public and consumers were told that this creation was, somehow, "better" than real eggs because it had no cholesterol in it! I wonder what people would say if they saw the results of a study done by Dr. Fred Kummernow of the University of Illinois at Urbana. He raised two litters of rats:

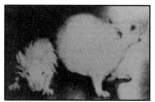

Weaned rats of the same age fed on fresh whole shell eggs (right) and artificial eggs, EggBeaters™, (left).

one on Egg Beaters, the other on real eggs. The rats on the real eggs thrived. The ones on Egg Beaters died before reaching adulthood.

This is the unfortunate reality of modern foods: they cannot support life. Each and every person I see with either heart disease, diabetes, cancer, or worse, has lived a life on technologically processed foods that were marketed as "healthy." Every elderly person I see with circulatory problems and atherosclerosis has used margarine and vegetable oils for their entire adult lives. They shunned the butter, cream, lard, tallow, and coconut oil of their youth as "unhealthy," believing the anti-fat rhetoric of modern nutrition. ◆ *The inevitable consequence of eating unnatural foods is sickness and death.* This is what Joe and his family have learned. Hopefully, you will learn it too in time to avoid an early visit from the Grim Reaper.

As you read this book, you will see that although heart disease has many causes, the main one today is a diet of processed, devitalized, sugar-laden "foods." If there is one thing you come away with from this book, I hope it is the knowledge that ◆ *real, whole, and natural food creates and sustains life*, and that imitation, fragmented, and new fangled food creates death and disease. You can start acting on this knowledge right now. Put down this book and go to your refrigerator. Throw out the margarine and vegetable oil spreads. Throw out the imitation cheeses, the "non-dairy" creamers, the mayonnaise and salad dressings made with sugar and oils, and the phony eggs. What should you replace them with? Keep reading.

Now, it is time to take a close look at the pioneering work of a man many have called "the Charles Darwin of nutrition," Dr. Weston Price. When you learn more about his incredible work, and what he found, you will better understand what creates good health and a healthy heart.

KEY POINTS TO REMEMBER

◆ *Heart disease was a rarity in Western countries until the late 1920s.*

◆ *The inevitable consequence of eating unnatural foods is sickness and death.*

◆ *As our food supply has "advanced," so have rates of chronic disease, including heart disease.*

◆ *Real, whole, and natural food creates and sustains life.*

CHAPTER TWO

There Was This Dentist...

As we enter the 21st century, one thing should be painfully clear after what we've learned in the last chapter: the 20th century exited with a crescendo of disease. ◆ *Despite our amazing scientific advances— television, movies, the space shuttle, walking on the moon, etc.—we have gotten nowhere when it comes to chronic disease.* Doctors cringe and cower when a patient with arthritis comes to see them. The same goes for people afflicted with Alzheimer's, Parkinson's, cancer, lupus, multiple sclerosis, and AIDS. Medical science, with all its technological wizardry (and overweening pride), has NO treatments or cures for any of these diseases and the rates for each of them keep climbing. When it comes to CVD, doctors may claim that they have reduced the mortality rates of people who have had heart attacks, but this is because science has the technology to keep people alive once they've had the heart attack. The **risk and incidence** of CVD, however, has only risen and worsened. ◆ *Despite the pushing of low fat/cholesterol diets, blood thinning drugs, polyunsaturated oils, and calorie counting, the 20th century has not made a dent in the rates of CVD.*

Things were not so bad back in 1930, but the situation was worsening enough to make one man take notice. Dr. Weston Price of Cleveland, Ohio, was a dentist in private practice who had a truly glorious and distinguished career. He had taught the science to thousands at dental schools, authored technical papers and textbooks, and headed an incredible study on the role of root canals in promoting diseases of various types. This last study was the subject of intense debate within the dental community with the more powerful minority winning out and eventually burying Dr. Price's massive research and disturbing conclusions. Basically, Dr. Price concluded that the bacteria that caused a tooth to decay were NOT eradicated fully by the root canal process, despite the dentist's best efforts to clean and disinfect the tooth. Price claimed that the bacteria remaining in the tooth continued to thrive and mutate into more virulent forms. These bacteria eventually found their way out of the mouth and invaded the body, causing various illnesses in susceptible people. Dr. Price called this the "Focal Infection Theory."

For those interested in reading more about this aspect of Dr. Price's work, the book, *Root Canal Cover-Up*, by Dr. George Meinig, DDS, is an excellent summary. It is available from The Price-Pottenger Nutrition Foundation, 1-800-FOODS4U or www.price-pottenger.org.

DR. PRICE'S NUTRITION STUDIES

Price noticed that his patients were suffering more and more chronic and degenerative diseases. He also noticed that his younger patients had increasingly deformed dental arches, crooked teeth, and cavities. This definitely concerned him, he had not seen such things ten or fifteen years ago. Why was it happening now? Price also noticed a strong correlation between dental health and physical health; a mouth full of cavities went hand in hand with a body either full of disease, or generalized weakness and susceptibility to disease. In Price's time, tuberculosis was the major infectious disease, the "White Scourge." He noticed that children were increasingly affected: the ones with the lousy teeth.

Dr. Price had heard rumors of native cultures where so-called primitive people lived happy lives, free of disease. He hit on an idea--why not go find these people and find out (1) if they really are healthy, and (2) if so, find out what they're doing to keep themselves healthy. Being rather well off financially, he and his wife started traveling around the world to remote locations. They were specifically looking for *healthy* peoples who had not been touched yet by civilization—at that time, such groups were still around.

Price's work is often criticized at this point for being biased. Critics claim that Price simply ignored native peoples that were not healthy, therefore, his data and conclusions about primitive diets are unfounded. These critics are missing the point and motivation for Dr. Price's work. Dr. Price was not interested in examining sick people because he'd seen enough of them in America. Price wanted to find *HEALTHY* people and find out what made them so, and if there were any patterns among these people. During his nine years of journeys, Price did indeed come across groups of primitives who were having problems for various reasons. Price noted these groups down, what appeared to be their difficulty, and then passed them over. Again, he was not interested in sick people. Price often found that the health problems were caused by food shortages (especially a lack of animal products), droughts, things people living off the land must face from time to time, or contact with white European civilization.

Dr. Price and his wife went just about everywhere in their journeys. They traveled to isolated villages in the Swiss alps, to cold and blustery islands off the coast of Scotland, to the Andes mountains in Peru, to several locations in Africa, to the Polynesian islands, to Australia and New Zealand, to the forests of northern Canada, and even to the Arctic Circle. In all, Price visited with fourteen groups of native peoples.

After gaining the trust of the village elders in the various places, Price did what came naturally; he counted cavities and physically examined them. Imagine his surprise to find, on average, less than 1% of tooth decay in all the peoples he visited! He also found that these people's teeth were perfectly straight and white, with high dental arches and well-formed facial features. There was something more astonishing, none of the peoples Price examined practiced any sort of dental hygiene; not one of his subjects had ever used a toothbrush! For example, when Price visited his first people, isolated Swiss mountain villagers, he noticed right away that the children's teeth were covered with a thin film of green slime, yet they had no tooth decay. What a difference this was from the children in Ohio!

Dr. Price also noticed that, in addition to their healthy teeth and gums, all the people he discovered were hardy and strong, despite the sometimes difficult living conditions they had to endure. Eskimo women, for example, gave birth to one healthy baby after another with little difficulty. Despite the Swiss children going barefoot in frigid streams, there had not been a single case of tuberculosis in any of them, despite exposure to TB. In general, Price found, in contrast to what he saw in America, no incidence of the very diseases that plague us "moderns" with our trash compactors and cellular phones, cancer, heart disease, diabetes, hemorrhoids, multiple sclerosis, Parkinson's, Alzheimer's, osteoporosis, chronic fatigue syndrome (it was called *neurasthenia* in Price's day), etc.

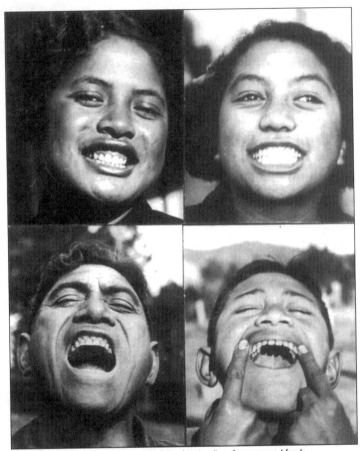

New Zealand Maori on traditional native diet of unprocessed foods.

Dr. Price also noticed another quality about the healthy primitives he found: they were happy. While depression was not a major problem in Price's day, it certainly is today, ask any psychiatrist. While certain natives sometimes fought with neighboring tribes, within their own groups, they were cheerful and optimistic and bounced back quickly from emotional setbacks. These people had no need for antidepressants.

Lest you think Dr. Price made all of this up, he was sure to take along with him one modern invention that would forever chronicle his research and startling conclusions--a camera. Dr. Price and his wife took pictures--

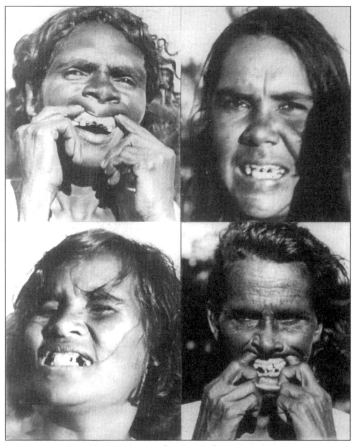

Australian Aborigines on a "modern diet" of processed foods.

18,000 of them. Many of the pictures are contained in Price's masterpiece *Nutrition and Physical Degeneration* (available from the PPNF website given earlier). The pictures show native peoples from all over the world smiling wide as the Mississippi river, their perfect teeth shining bright.

WHAT THE PEOPLE ATE

Dr. Price, in addition to examining the natives, also gathered considerable data about their distinctive cultures and customs, and these descriptions fill many of the pages of his book. Price took great care to observe what these people were eating for he suspected the key to good health and good teeth was in good food. He was surprised to find that, depending on the people in question and where they lived, each group ate very differently from the other. For example, the Swiss mountain villagers subsisted primarily on unpasteurized and cultured dairy products, especially butter and cheese. Rye also formed an integral part of their diet. Occasionally, they ate meat (beef) as cows in their herds got older. Small amounts of bone broths, vegetables and berries rounded out the diet. Due to the high altitude, not much vegetation grew. The villagers would eat what they could in the short summer months, and pickle what was left over for the winter. The main foods, however, were full fat cheese, butter, and rye bread.

Gaelic fisher people of the Outer Hebrides ate no dairy products, but instead had their fill of cod and other sea foods, especially shellfish (when in season). Due to the poor soil, the only grain that could grow was oat, and it formed a major part of the diet. A traditional dish, one considered very important for growing children and expectant mothers, was cod's head stuffed with oats and mashed fish liver. Again, due to the extremely inhospitable climate, fruits and vegetables grew sparsely. Price noted that a young Gaelic girl reeled in puzzlement when offered an apple; she had never seen one!

Eskimo, or Inuit, ate a diet of almost 100% animal products with hefty amounts of fish. Walrus and seal, and other marine mammals also formed an integral part of the diet. Blubber (fat) was consumed with relish. Inuit would gather nuts, berries, and some grasses during the short summer months, but their diet was basically all meat and fat. Price noted that the Inuit would usually ferment their meat before eating it. That is, they would bury it and allow it to slightly putrefy before consuming it. Don't be disgusted. Whenever you eat yogurt, you're eating a similar food product, made in the same way by beneficial lactic acid bacteria. Inuit would also eat the partially digested grasses of caribou by cutting open their stomachs and intestines.

The Maori of New Zealand, along with other South sea islanders, consumed sea food of every sort—fish, shark, octopus, sea worms, shellfish—along with fatty pork and a wide variety of plant foods including coconut and fruit.

African cattle-keeping tribes like the Masai consumed virtually no plant foods at all, just beef, raw milk, organ meats, and blood (in times of drought).

The Dinkas of the Sudan, whom Price claimed were the healthiest of all the African tribes he studied, ate a combination of fermented whole grains with fish, along with smaller amounts of red meat, vegetables, and fruit. The Bantu, on the other hand, the least hardy of the African tribes studied, were primarily agriculturists. Their diet consisted mostly of beans, squash, corn, millet, vegetables, and fruits, with small amounts of milk and meat. Price never found a totally vegetarian culture. Modern anthropological data support this: all cultures and peoples show a preference for animal foods and animal fat (Abrams, "The Preference for ...").

Hunter-gatherer peoples in Northern Canada, the Florida Everglades, the Amazon, and Australia, consumed game animals of all types, especially the organ meats, and a variety of grains, legumes, tubers, vegetables, and fruits when available.

Price noted that all peoples, except the Inuit, consumed insects and their larvae. Obviously in more tropical areas, insects formed a more integral part of the diet. "The natives of Africa know that certain insects are very rich in special food values at certain seasons, also that their eggs are valuable foods. A fly that hatches in enormous quantities in Lake Victoria is gathered and used fresh and dried for storage. They also use ant eggs and ants." Bees, wasps, dragonflies, beetles, crickets, cicadas, moths, and termites were consumed with zest also, particularly in Africa.

Price also noted that all cultures consumed fermented foods each day. Foods such as cheese, cultured butter, yogurt, or fermented grain drinks like kaffir beer (made from millet) in Africa, or fermented fish as with the Inuit, were an important part of native diets.

Curiously, all native peoples studied made great efforts to obtain seafood, especially fish roe which was consumed "so that we will have healthy children." Even mountain dwelling peoples would make semiannual trips to the sea to bring back seaweeds, fish eggs, and dried fish. Shrimp, rich in both cholesterol and vitamin D, was a standard food in many places, from Africa to the Orient.

The last major feature of native diets that Price found was that they were rich in fat, especially animal fat. Whether from insects, eggs, fish, game animals, or domesticated herds, primitive peoples knew that they would get sick if they did not consume enough fat. Explorers besides Dr. Price have also found this to be true. For example, anthropologist Vilhjalmur Stefansson, who lived for years among the Inuit and Northern Canadian Indians, specifically noted how the Indians would go out of their way to hunt down older male caribou for they carried a 50 pound slab of back fat. When such animals were unavailable and Indians were forced to subsist on rabbits, a very lean animal, diarrhea and hunger would set in after about a week. The human body needs saturated fat to properly utilize essential fatty acids. Saturated animal fats contain high amounts of the fat soluble vitamins needed to assimilate proteins and minerals, as well as beneficial fatty acids with antimicrobial properties.

Of course, the foods that Price's subjects ate were natural and unprocessed. Their foods did not contain preservatives, additives, or colorings. They did not contain added sugar (though, when available, natural sweets like honey and maple syrup were eaten in moderation). They did not contain white flour or canned foods. Their milk products were not pasteurized, homogenized, or low fat. The animal and plant foods consumed were raised and grown on pesticide-free soil and were not given growth hormones or antibiotics. In short, these people always ate organic.

WHAT THE SAMPLES SHOWED

Dr. Price was eager to chemically analyze the various foods these primitives ate. He was careful to obtain preserved samples of all types for analysis. Basically, ◆ *the diets of these healthy peoples contained 10 times the amount of fat-soluble vitamins, and at least 4 times the amount of calcium, other minerals, and water soluble vitamins than Western diets at that time.* No wonder these people were so healthy!

Because of the consumption of fermented and raw foods (including raw animal products), Price noted that native diets were rich in enzymes. Enzymes assist in the digestion of cooked foods.

Price noted that all peoples had a predilection and dietary pull towards foods rich in the fat-soluble vitamins. Price considered butter from pasture-fed cows, rich in these vitamins as well as minerals, to be the premiere health food. Fat-soluble vitamins are found in fats of animal origin, like butter, cream, lard, and tallow.

I know what some of you are thinking: "All these foods are the very ones I've been told are bad for my health and my heart!" It is true, Dr. Price's research and conclusions are disturbing to modern nutritionists because they stand in stark contrast to their gospel of lean meat, grains, vegetables, fruit, and skim milk. As we shall see, however, ◆ *the low fat diet pushed by most of modern nutrition is a prescription for ill health.*

To dispel a common myth about native peoples, they did live long lives. Price took numerous photos of healthy primitives with heads full of gray hair. While we don't know exactly how old they were since they did not have calendars, they were, by all appearances, well past 60. The Aborigines, for example, had a special society of the elderly. Obviously, if there were no old people among them, they would have had no need for such a group. Stefansson also reported great longevity among the Inuit. It is true that death rates at younger ages were higher among some groups, but these mortalities were from the dangerous life-style these people lived, not from their diet. When you live in the Arctic Circle, for example, constantly fighting the elements, polar bears, ice flows, and leopard seals, you run the risk of an early death.

Another common misconception that modern nutrition holds towards native peoples and their high meat and fat diets is that they suffered from all sorts of degenerative diseases, especially osteoporosis and heart disease. The facts, however, do not support these contentions. Despite some studies done in the past few decades that tried to show the high rates of osteoporosis among the Inuit were due to their high protein diet, other studies have shown no such thing. The work of Dr. Herta Spencer and Dr. Lois Kramer conclusively proved that the protein/calcium loss theory was nonsense. As it turns out, the negative studies on the Eskimo were done, not on Inuit following their traditional diet, but among modernized Inuit who had adopted modern eating habits and alcohol. Alcoholism is a major factor in bone loss. Certainly, Dr. Price would have noted that bone loss was a problem if it had been, especially since he was examining teeth which are made of calcium, but he did not. While in Switzerland, Price got permission to dig up skeletal remains of some villagers; the bones were sturdy and strong. There are pictures in Price's book of these bones (and skulls showing mouths of perfect teeth free of decay). Price (and other researchers after him whom we'll discuss in chapter four) found no incidence of any major diseases, including heart disease.

This is not to say that native peoples did not have ANY problems for such is certainly not the case. Price learned of native remedies for a host of minor ills such as headaches, colds, wounds, and burns. As far as degenerative diseases go, he found nothing.

This brings up the other major finding of Dr. Price's research--the effects of a modern diet on native peoples. To this, let us now turn.

THE ROOTS OF DISEASE

When Dr. Price visited the various primitive groups, he noted that white European civilization had begun making inroads into the areas where they lived. Some of the native peoples opted to leave and move into areas where it was more "modern." Dr. Price also had the opportunity to compare white colonialists who were living alongside, or close to, the native peoples he was studying. What he found was what he thought he would find—disease and dental decay.

When people read *Nutrition* and *Physical Degeneration*, it often changes their lives because not only does it describe how healthy people look, feel, and eat, it also shows in painful detail what happens to those people when they abandon their native eating patterns and adopt what I like to call "*haole* food." *Haole* is the Hawaiian word for "white man" (I might as well blame my own race!). The pictures Price took of natives and moderns on what Price disdainfully called "the displacing foods of modern commerce" are horrifying and stand in stark contrast to the pictures next to them of healthy, smiling natives. Nutrition writer and Price enthusiast, Sally Fallon, explains:

> "His photographs capture the suffering caused by these foodstuffs—
> chiefly rampant tooth decay. Even more startling, they show the
> change in facial development that occurred with modernization.
> Parents who had changed their diets gave birth to children who
> no longer exhibited the tribal patterns. Their faces were more
> narrow, their teeth crowded, their nostrils pinched. These faces
> do not beam with optimism, like those of their healthy ancestors.
> The photographs of Dr. Weston Price demonstrate with great
> clarity that the 'displacing foods of modern commerce' do not
> provide sufficient nutrients to allow the body to reach its full
> genetic potential—neither the complete development of the
> bones in the body and the head, nor the fullest expressions
> of the various systems that allow humankind to function at
> optimal levels—immune system, nervous system, digestion,
> and reproduction." ("Nasty, Brutish, and Short?", 8).

And what were the offending foods that these unfortunate people consumed? Why everything you find on your grocer's shelves-- sugar, white flour, jams, jellies, cookies, condensed milk, canned vegetables, pastries, refined grain products, margarine, and vegetable oils.

Price noted in several places that where modern foods had displaced traditional ones, suicide rates from dental caries were high. As most of us know, dental pain can be excruciating. With no drugs to ease their pain, and no dentist around to pull the dying tooth, people took their own lives to escape the torture.

White Europeans who lived in Africa had to leave periodically for health reasons. Children born there had to be sent away several times during their youth in order to survive. Such was the "hardy" effect of modern foods on these people. Native Africans, of course, had no such problems as long as they stayed on their native diets.

As I noted earlier, the major infectious disease at Price's time was tuberculosis, the White Scourge. Price took several photographs of children, usually the children of either Europeans or natives who had adopted the modern foods before their children were born. They are disturbing in their depictions of suffering. Some of the children were too sick to be moved to better lighting for photographing. Others had pus visibly draining from their lymph glands and abscessed teeth. Invariably, ◆ *parents and children who had adopted modern foods were highly susceptible to tuberculosis and other degenerative diseases.*

The native Hawaiians are a tragic example of this shift. Price did visit the Hawaiian islands on his journeys. He, of course, noted that Hawaiians who ate their traditional diet of coconut, fish, taro, sweet potatoes, and fresh fruits were healthy and strong. Today, however, the health of native Hawaiians is frightening. Obesity and diabetes are rampant. Because canned meats with nitrates in them are popular there, rates of stomach cancer are high (nitrates convert into carcinogens in the stomach—vitamin C halts the conversion). Hawaiians today eat their fair share of sugar, soft drinks, vegetable oils, macaroni salad, white flour, and white rice. Coconut is sometimes eaten, but usually as part of a sugary snack. High blood pressure and heart attacks are common. Rates of Alzheimer's are elevated as well. Such is the effect of processed foods on a beautiful race of people.

In the last decade or so, however, a diet was proposed called the Hawaii Diet. Though it is a little low in fat for my tastes, it advocates a full return to traditional eating patterns: fish, taro, sweet potatoes, fresh fruit and vegetables, and, occasionally, pork (wild boar and feral pig are native to the islands). Specifically avoided are white rice, sugar, Spam, and processed foods in general. The change is dramatic: people lose weight, they have more energy, and their health problems dissipate or become more manageable. Their teeth invariably improve as well.

Price noticed this pattern also. If a native abandoned his ancestral eating habits in favor of modern foods, ill health and dental caries followed. If that same person switched back to the original eating pattern, however, health returned and the progression of dental decay stopped and reversed itself. This is perhaps the most uplifting aspect of Price's work: one can always reverse the trend; there is always hope.

Price accurately and ominously predicted that as Western man consumed more refined sugar and substituted vegetable oils for animal fats, disease would increase and reproduction would be more difficult. Today, some 25% of Western couples are infertile, and rates of cancer, diabetes, and heart disease have skyrocketed. Price was truly a modern Cassandra of Troy—prophesying the truth, but with no one listening.

A RETURN TO SANITY, PLEASE?

For many decades, Price's work has been buried and forgotten. Due to the efforts of the Price-Pottenger Nutrition Foundation and the Weston A. Price Foundation, however, and the republication of Price's book for the public, that is fortunately starting to change. Several prominent nutritional doctors have traced their philosophical heritages back to Weston Price and his work. Abram Hoffer, founder and developer of orthomolecular psychiatry, Jonathan Wright, noted author, Alan Gaby, medical columnist, Melvyn Werbach, nutritional author, and other medical doctors all sing the praises of this ingenious dentist. Nutritional anthropologist, H. Leon Abrams, associate professor emeritus at the University System of Georgia and author of over 200 papers and eight books, points to Price as a "giant, ahead of his time with a message relevant to us all."

Price's conclusions and recommendations were shocking for his time. He advocated a return to breast feeding when such a practice was discouraged by Western medicine. He urged parents to give their children cod liver oil every day. He considered fresh butter to be the supreme health food. He warned against pesticides, herbicides, preservatives, colorings, refined sugars, vegetable oils, in short, all the things that modern nutrition and agriculture have embraced and promoted the last few decades. Price believed that margarine was a demonic creation. Let me tell you, with recommendations like these, he was REALLY unpopular! But the result of his research speaks for itself.

Knowing that his data flatly contradicts virtually everything that "politically correct" nutrition holds, it is common to find his work belittled. If Price's studies are accurate, then the low-fat school must go the way of all flesh: into the graveyard. It is typical, therefore, for critics to say things like Price only superficially examined the peoples he encountered and made simplistic conclusions about their health. Price is also accused of ignoring the nutritional deficiencies of the peoples he studied, as well as their high rates of infant mortality. Its also asserted that the modern foods that Price argued were these peoples' downfall were actually "wholesome," but the primitive peoples overconsumed too much of them and didn't "balance" their diets correctly, hence their high rates of disease after adopting modern food stuffs. Critics also claim that malnourished people usually don't have dental problems, so it is immaterial that the natives Price photographed had perfect teeth, or that the modernized ones had poor ones. Another recent objection to surface is that Dr. Price's research is irrelevant to us today because it is 70 years old and therefore not current.

It is truly amazing how far some "experts" will go to defend the processed food industry and shaky nutritional hypotheses! Even a cursory look at Price's book will tell any rational person that Price did not "superficially examine" the people he studied. The detail about native customs, eating habits, and history of the various areas argues against any accusations of superficiality. Additionally, Price was a physician with many years of experience; it is ludicrous to claim that he would make a "superficial examination" and reach "simplistic conclusions" about peoples' health. If there were nutritional deficiencies, he would have noted them down, but no such descriptions exist for the simple reason that *no such deficiencies existed.* We know this to be true for, if we examine the modern descendants of Price's subjects, we find that they enjoy robust health and freedom from both dental caries and more chronic diseases, IF they have not abandoned their native diets.

It is true that high infant mortality rates existed, but only AFTER exposure to and adoption of the white European way of life. Further, if the foods of modern commerce were so wholesome, then they would have provided the nutrients within them to avert death, dental decay, and disease in the person who ate them, regardless of how they ingested them. Claims of "unbalanced diets" of modern foods is plain old double-talk that does not stand the test of logic.

The last claim about dental conditions not being related to the body's nutritional state is an out and out lie. Numerous researchers have noted the clear and obvious connection between dental and bodily health. They all assert without hesitation that the health of the body is reflected quite accurately in the health of the teeth (Abrams, "Vegetarianism" 72; Diorio, et. al. 856-865; Menaker and Navia 680-687).

Finally, Price's findings are most certainly relevant today. Price did not theorize about human nutrition, he made observations of healthy peoples and then drew general conclusions from those peoples' diets. Since the human genome has not significantly changed in 70 years, those observations and conclusions are still pertinent today.

DR. PRICE'S MESSAGE

The obvious conclusion of Price's research is that ◆ *for humanity to survive, it must eat better.* The foods it consumes must be whole, fresh, and unprocessed. More and more, people are beginning to see this and have been changing their eating patterns. For the majority, however, the continuation of negative dietary habits will inevitably lead to decreased vitality, unhealthy children, in short, the degeneration of the human race. In this world of survival of the fittest, we need to take every opportunity to bolster our position or we risk going the way of the dodo bird: into extinction. Hopefully, through this book, you'll take the opportunity I'm giving you to improve and strengthen, not just your heart, but your entire body and mind.

Besides, eating whole foods tastes good! The first happy lesson to be gleaned from traditional diets and Price's work is that good food can and should taste good. Its OK to saute vegetables and meats with butter. Its OK to consume whole milk, meat with its fat, eggs, shrimp and lobster, and liver with onions and bacon. Its OK and healthy to eat homemade soups made from gelatin-rich bone broths and sauces made from drippings and cream.

Eating whole foods is good for the environment as well. The building blocks of a whole foods diet are pesticide-free plant foods raised on naturally enriched soils, and healthy animals that live free to graze and manure the paddocks of their farms, as opposed to standing in cramped stalls, never seeing sunlight, being fed soybeans and corn meal, and being shot up with steroids and antibiotics.

Eating whole foods is better for the economy as well. Organic foods are usually raised by small farms. Each time you buy an organically raised plant or animal product, you are helping someone to earn a living. Isn't that preferable to giving your money to a multinational food company that mass produces its product, not caring about the health of the soil, the planet, the animals, or ourselves?

Finally, ◆ *eating whole foods is healthier.* We humans evolved eating certain food stuffs in certain ways. You did not see a caveman trimming the fat off of his meat—he ate the whole thing. You did not see a Swiss Alps villager eating low fat cheese—she ate the whole thing. You did not see Maori fishermen avoiding shellfish for fear of cholesterol—they ate the whole thing. Foods are packaged in ways that Nature intended: they contain all the nutrients within themselves for optimal assimilation by our bodies. Eating whole foods insures us the highest amount of nutrients food has to offer. Tampering with them is ill advised.

KEY POINTS TO REMEMBER

◆ *Despite our amazing scientific advances—television, movies, the space shuttle, walking on the moon, etc.—we have gotten nowhere when it comes to chronic disease.*

◆ *Despite the pushing of low fat/cholesterol diets, blood thinning drugs, polyunsaturated oils, and calorie counting, the 20th century has not made a dent in the rates of CVD.*

◆ *The diets of these healthy peoples contained 10 times the amount of vitamins A and D, and at least 4 times the amount of calcium and other minerals than American diets at that time.*

◆ *Parents and children who had adopted haole food were highly susceptible to tuberculosis and other degenerative diseases.*

◆ *For humanity to survive, it must eat better.*

◆ *Eating whole foods is healthier.*

◆ *The low fat diet pushed by most of modern nutrition is a prescription for ill health.*

CHAPTER THREE

Big Fat Lies

The current theory offered to explain how heart disease has risen to become the Western world's number one killer is called the **Lipid Hypothesis.** Basically, this theory states that saturated fats and cholesterol clog the arteries, leading to atherosclerosis, heart disease, and an ever-increasing assortment of serious illnesses, most notably cancer. According to this theory, the main reason why heart disease and cancer rates have skyrocketed in this century is because people have been eating more and more saturated fat and cholesterol-rich foods. The solution to heart disease (and cancer) is to simply reduce our consumption of such foods, replacing them with more complex carbohydrates, fruits, vegetables, legumes, and unsaturated fats, especially polyunsaturated ones which have been shown to reduce serum cholesterol levels. Traditional foods like butter, cream, lard, meats, and eggs have been blamed for horrible diseases, especially heart disease. Eliminate them, say the experts, and your risk for heart disease will drop drastically. Diets low in fat are also urged by some health professionals for people with current heart conditions or high blood cholesterol levels. A brief scan of nutrition books, both for the professional and the lay person, well illustrates the philosophy of the Lipid Hypothesis.

While most people are aware that cholesterol is a culprit in heart disease, the average American continues to consume about 175 pounds of meat, 234 eggs, about 15 pounds of margarine and butter, and almost 18 pounds of ice cream annually, while the heart struggles to pump blood through arteries accumulating cholesterol deposits at a rate of 1 to 2 percent per year. . . Year after year, study after study, cholesterol's role as a promoter of CVD has been, and continues to be, confirmed. The risk of developing cardiovascular disease is directly related to serum cholesterol levels. As cholesterol rises above 200 mg/dl, CVD rates climb proportionately. A direct correlation exists between the incidence of CVD in a particular group, blood cholesterol levels, and the amount of fatty foods of animal origin in the diet...The link between dietary fat and cardiovascular disease (CVD) is well-documented (Garrison & Somer 342-343, 360).

We have gradually increased our intake of butter, milk, other dairy products and eggs. The proportion of calories from fat has increased from a national figure of 30 percent in 1910 to over 40 percent [with a corresponding increase in heart disease] (Stamler 3).

Coronary heart disease is a twentieth-century phenomenon—and so is the emphasis on animal products in our diet. In the early 1900's, coronary heart disease was a comparatively rare illness...The rise of coronary heart disease in the United States [and other Western countries] paralleled the changes in the U.S. dietary habits. As the consumption of animal fat and cholesterol began to rise during this century, so did the incidence of coronary heart disease. People in most of the world...have never increased their consumption of animal products. In these countries, coronary heart disease is still a rare illness (Ornish 144-145).

It is very common in nutritional medicine books to see low fat diet/low cholesterol diets recommended for hypertension and CVD. Such diets are also urged for "cancer prevention" and improved vitality and well being. All of the major health and nutritional organizations in the Western world embrace and promote the Lipid Hypothesis and its twin, the Cholesterol Hypothesis. Along with these two goes another theory about high and low density lipoproteins (or HDL and LDL, respectively). While we'll look at this theory by itself later in this chapter, what you need to know now is that, according to this theory, higher levels of HDL's translate to a decreased rate and risk for heart disease, while higher levels of LDL's translate to the exact opposite. It is routine for people having a general check-up to have their serum cholesterol levels checked, as well as their ratio of HDL's to LDL's. A cholesterol reading over 200 mg/dl is viewed as a risk for CVD.

In general, although other factors such as smoking and stress are acknowledged, modern medical and nutritional thought tends to blame CVD on a diet rich in saturated fats and cholesterol.

The Lipid Hypothesis has been a boon for many industries, especially the pharmaceutical and food processing ones which make a very brisk dollar on cholesterol-lowering drugs and low-fat/cholesterol processed foods. In America right now, a margarine derived from pine tree sterols is about to hit the market; the plant sterols in it lower cholesterol levels. Speaking of margarine, the other major benefactor of the Lipid Hypothesis has been the vegetable oil and shortening industry. Since most vegetable oils are high in polyunsaturated fatty acids (or PUFA's, discussed below), and since PUFA's lower serum cholesterol levels, corn, safflower, soybean, and in some countries canola, oils have been heavily marketed to the public. For example, a popular brand of corn oil in America was advertised for years in popular and professional magazines as "good for your heart" and labeled a "cholesterol depressant" (Fallon & Enig "Oiling," 3).

Since margarine is manufactured from vegetable oils, it was also heavily promoted to the public and medical profession as being more "heart healthy" than butter or lard. To this day, companies will conspicuously label a product as "Low In Fat," "Fat-Free," or "Cholesterol-Free" to enhance sales. In the mind of the public, the words "cholesterol" and "fat" have become synonymous with disease, while "low fat, low cholesterol" have become synonymous with health.

An indirect result of the Lipid Hypothesis has been an increasing number of people embracing vegetarianism. Since saturated fat is found primarily in animal foods, and since cholesterol is only found in animal foods, many have eliminated animal products from their diets in the belief that it is healthier for them. Health food companies that manufacture vegetable replacement foods, such as soy milk and imitation chicken, beef, or cheese made from soybeans or other vegetable proteins, have benefited as well. As a matter of fact, a whole industry of processed "health" foods has mushroomed in the last twenty years. Products include eggless mayonnaise made from assorted vegetable oils, egg replacer products made from vegetable proteins and oils, and an array of foods manufactured from organically raised plant foods.

Of course, a bevy of scientific studies have been done that supposedly prove the Lipid Hypothesis and that eliminating saturated fats is a good idea. The media, of course, reports these studies to the public who, of course, believe them.

Unfortunately, the Lipid Hypothesis has never been proven to be true. All of you should have seen from the last chapter that ◆ *Dr. Price's studies of real people and what they actually ate, show that a high intake of saturated fat produced robust health.* There have always been scientific detractors from the Lipid Hypothesis, some very vocal in fact, but their minority views never seem to get much attention, either from the medical or media communities. Nevertheless, the evidence against the Lipid Hypothesis, as well as its companions, the Cholesterol and HDL/LDL theories, is there and deserves our attention. Before we get into this, however, we need to clarify a few things about lipids, or FATS, so we'll all know what we're talking about.

LOTS OF LIPIDS

As you might have noticed in reading the excerpt from Garrison and Somer above, there is an unfortunate tendency for nutrition writers to mix different kinds of fats together, treating them as if they were all the same. In the passage above, the authors list meat, milk, eggs, butter, margarine, and ice cream in the same breath. This creates the impression to the reader that one fat is the same as another fat. This is false. The error is repeated time and time again by researchers who hold to the Lipid Hypothesis. At the onset, then, you must always remember that there are different types of fat, each with a mode of action different from the other. Lipid biochemistry is a complicated field, but anyone can understand the basics. Let's define our terms.

Fatty acids are chains of carbon and hydrogen atoms, some short, some long depending on the one in question. They are placed into three groups: **saturated (SFA), monounsaturated (MUFA), and polyunsaturated (PUFA).** The number of available carbon bonds in the fatty acid molecule is what determines its degree of saturation. If all of the carbon bonds in a fatty acid are full and occupied by hydrogen atoms, it is *saturated.* If two carbon atoms are double-bonded to each other, therefore lacking two hydrogen atoms, it is *monounsaturated. All fats, whether of animal or vegetable origin, are blends of these three types of fatty acids but with one type usually predominating, depending on the food in question.*

28

Saturated fats predominate principally in an˙
and coconut oils are noted plant sources. Monoᴜ
in nuts, avocados, olive oil, and some animal fats (espᴇ
unsaturated fats mostly make up vegetable fat, but appreciaʋ
are found in fish oils and chicken skin. Important exceptions to thᵢ
commercially-raised animals that have been fed a high vegetable diet.
The best example of this is a commercially-raised turkey. This meat
source usually has dry flesh and goes bad quickly in the refrigerator; the
result of too many polyunsaturates in its body.

It should be noted here that ◆ *the more a fat is saturated, the more
stable it is chemically.* Saturated and monounsaturated fats do not go
rancid easily if stored properly. Likewise, these fats are more stable under heat, making them ideal for cooking. Polyunsaturated fats, however, especially those of vegetable origin, are not as stable and go rancid
more quickly, even in the body. Rancid oils breed one thing: cancer-
causing and tissue damaging free radicals. While some polyunsaturated
fats are needed by the body, they should not exceed 5% of your total
caloric intake due to this problem. Ironically, it is the polyunsaturates
that have been urged by health experts for the last 50 years. And as
people have consumed more of them, certain health problems, like heart
disease, have escalated.

There are two types of polyunsaturated fatty acids that are vital for
our health: omega 3's and omega 6's. These are also known as the *essential
fatty acids* (EFA's) and, like vitamins and minerals, must be gotten from
our food. The body manufactures *prostaglandins* from certain EFA's. Prostaglandins are localized tissue hormones that appear to regulate numerous chemical activities in our cells. In times past, humans consumed a
balance of omega 3's (found in fish, walnuts, eggs, flax oil, dark green
leafy vegetables, and some whole grains) and omega 6's (found principally in plant foods), and this is as it should be as both are equally important. When there is an overabundance of omega 6's in the diet, however,
our body's ability to absorb and utilize the omega 3's is inhibited. This
causes a host of undesirable reactions including sexual and immune dysfunction, and increased cancer risk (Fallon, Enig, & Connolly 10). This
is something that most modern lipid researchers, especially those wedded
to the Lipid Hypothesis, either overlook or do not know.

There is another type of "fat" that is produced during chemical
processing called a *trans-fatty acid* (TFA). The major way that trans-fats
are produced is by forcing hydrogen atoms into a vegetable oil that has

had a nickel catalyst added to it. In other words, **hydrogenation** makes a liquid lipid (vegetable oil) solid through chemical tampering. Although the finished product looks like a saturated fat (also solid), its chemical structure is very different. These are unnatural fats that our bodies cannot utilize properly because of that chemical structure. These fake fats are found in margarine, "vegetable oil spreads," shortening, processed vegetable oils, and canola oil, as well as any foods made with them. As we shall see, ◆ *it is mostly trans-fatty acid consumption, and not saturated fat consumption, that is strongly correlated with increased cancer and cardiovascular disease.*

Cholesterol is a heavy weight molecule, actually an alcohol or sterol. It is a slippery substance that moves at a high rate of speed through the body. It is found in every cell membrane. It is also the substrate used by the body to manufacture several hormones (e.g., adrenaline and progesterone). It is also an antioxidant that the body uses to repair damaged tissues, including weakened arteries.

Although the foregoing discussion is by no means complete, it is enough to give you some basic knowledge in lipids. This should help you to understand this chapter more.

THE HISTORY OF THE LIPID HYPOTHESIS

As mentioned earlier, heart disease and deaths from myocardial infarction (MI), a massive blood clot leading to death of the heart muscle, were extremely rare at the turn of the century. This rarity continued up until the late 1920s. Then, things started to change for the worse. Doctors who had never even seen a heart attack patient their entire careers, now began seeing them with increased frequency. By the 1950s, heart disease and MI's accounted for about 30% of all deaths in Western countries. That figure has risen steadily and now holds at about 45%. In just five or six decades, a once rare condition grew to become our number one killer.

Scientists and doctors in the 1950s were grappling with this problem, trying to figure out what had caused the dramatic rise. In 1954, a young researcher named David Kritchevsky published a paper describing the effects of feeding cholesterol to rabbits. The young Russian mixed the substance with rabbit chow. He noted that the rabbits developed arterial plaque, i.e., atherosclerosis. The studies were actually repeats of experiments carried out decades before, also in Russia, in which cholesterol fed to rabbits resulted in clogged arteries and heart problems.

Later in 1954, Kritchevsky published another paper demonstrating that PUFA's in the diet could lower blood cholesterol levels. These two studies attracted immediate attention for they lent support to a theory that had developed to explain the rise of CVD: that saturated fats and cholesterol from animal products raise cholesterol levels in the blood, leading to cholesterol and fat deposits in the arteries. Thus, the Lipid Hypothesis was born.

In 1956, the American Heart Association (AHA) held a nationally-televised fund-raiser to officially present the Lipid Hypothesis to the public and to kick-off the AHA's "Prudent Diet." The Prudent Diet called for the replacement of margarine for butter, skinless chicken for beef, cold cereal and toast for bacon and eggs, low-fat or skim milk for whole milk and cream, and corn oil for tallow and lard. The Master of Ceremonies interviewed doctors who endorsed the Lipid Hypothesis, Irving Page and Jeremiah Stamler, among others. Someone else interviewed was Dr. Paul Dudley White. When pressed to endorse the Lipid Hypothesis and the Prudent Diet, White surprisingly retorted: "See here, I began my practice as a cardiologist in 1921 and I never saw an MI patient until 1928. Back in the MI-free days before 1920, the fats were butter and lard, and I think that we would all benefit from the kind of diet that we had at a time when no one had ever heard the word 'corn' oil" (Fallon & Enig "Oiling" 3).

Despite this glitch, the televised campaign was a success in terms of public acceptance. On the surface, it appeared that the theory was true as it was so simple: if you eat more fat and cholesterol, then more will clog your arteries. A number of researchers appeared in support of the Lipid Hypothesis. One of the most famous was Ancel Keys. Keys headed up the massive Seven Countries Study where he and his colleagues analyzed the diets of 12,000 men in seven countries. They concluded that the men who ate the most fat had the highest rates of CVD, while the men who ate the least had the lowest rates of CVD. This was odd as Keys had, in 1956, suggested in a published paper that the increasing use of hydrogenated vegetable oils might be the underlying cause of CVD (Keys, "Diet & Development"). Other studies in later years (discussed below) were undertaken to prove the Lipid Hypothesis.

One of the more interesting studies was orchestrated by Dr. Norman Jolliffe, Director of the Nutrition Bureau of the New York Health Department. He organized the Anti-Coronary Club in 1957, in which selected businessmen, ranging in age from 40-59 years were placed on the AHA's Prudent Diet. Club members followed the Diet religiously. They were to be compared to another group of businessmen who ate eggs and bacon for breakfast, used butter, and ate meat three times a day. Jolliffe, an overweight diabetic confined to a wheelchair, was confident, along with the other Lipid Hypothesis supporters, that the "Prudent" group would fare much better than the "non-Prudent" group.

In 1966, the results of the study were published in the *Journal of the American Medical Association* (Cristakis 129-135). Although the Prudent Diet men had slightly lower serum cholesterol levels than the non-Prudent group (220 vs. 250), ***there were eight deaths from heart disease in the Prudent group and none in the non-Prudent group!*** Despite this negative study, the Lipid Hypothesis kept marching on. Oh, and Dr. Jolliffe? He died of a vascular thrombosis in 1961. Apparently, the Prudent Diet was not able to save him either (Fallon & Enig "Oiling" 4).

Deaths from heart attacks seemed to strike other supporters of the Lipid Hypothesis as well. For example, Dr. Irving Page, on the AHA panel in the 1956 broadcast, who wanted to organize a more extensive trial to prove the Prudent Diet's effectiveness after the dismal results of Jolliffe's "Anti-Coronary Club" experiment, also died of a heart attack. Page's planned dietary experiment was abandoned in silence.

Nevertheless, the Lipid Hypothesis, despite the initial resistance from the American Medical Association, took off and entrenched itself in the minds of Western researchers. Things were helped along by slick advertising campaigns carried out by vegetable oil and margarine companies in which doctors such as Frederick Stare of Harvard University endorsed new fangled products and belittled traditional animal fats and cholesterol-containing foods.

By the 1970s, the American Medical Association, the American Dietetics Association, the National Academy of Sciences (USA), and the National Heart, Lung, and Blood Institute (USA) had endorsed the Lipid Hypothesis and called for Americans, and by extension all Westerners, to throw away butter, cream, lard, and fatty meats and sausages, and embrace corn oil, margarine, imitation eggs, skim milk, lean meats, and more plant foods. A dietary committee in America headed by Senator George McGovern in the 1970s, urged PUFA consumption and elimination of animal fats. American doctors received a "Cholesterol Education Kit" in the 1980s in which cholesterol screening was encouraged, as well as the use of cholesterol-lowering drugs and margarine.

DISSENTING VOICES

Dr. White's pleas in 1956 went unheard at the time, but he had brought up a telling point: how could the Lipid Hypothesis possibly be true if, ◆ *in times when heart disease and MI's were rare, people consumed plenty of animal fats, namely, butter and lard? Indeed, how could it be true?* One would expect to see the same high rates of CVD in those who ate a lot of animal fats, like the people Dr. Price studied, but such was not the case. Several nutrition researchers noted the same thing and began to publish their objections.

Dr. Fred Kummerow of the University of Illinois at Urbana had conducted studies in the early 1970s showing that the consumption of trans fatty acids in margarine and processed vegetable oils caused increased rates of heart disease in pigs ("Effects of Isomeric Fats..." 151-180). Kummerow also authored the paper showing that imitation eggs could not support life. Kummerow also wrote a moving and impassioned letter against the Lipid Hypothesis and submitted it to the US Senate Committee on Nutrition and Human Needs in the early 1970s. Kummerow specifically urged a return to traditional foods and fats, the very ones demonized by the Lipid Hypothesis (and the Senate Committee)--butter, cream, eggs, milk, lard, and tallow. Kummerow's papers, rat pictures, and letter were summarily ignored and buried.

Kummerow also discovered the result of holding an unpopular minority opinion: his subsequent applications for research funding in nutritional biochemistry were all turned down. Had it not been for a private endowment, he would have been unable to continue his work.

I recently interviewed the venerable Kummerow, who is still doing research at the University of Illinois. He told me an interesting story about his damning paper on imitation eggs. "I originally submitted it to the *Journal of the American Medical Association [JAMA]*, but the assistant editor at the time rejected it and advised me to submit it instead to *Pediatrics,* a lesser journal also owned by the American Medical Association. *Pediatrics* published the paper and the photos. I think I know why the editor turned the article down; the following issue of *JAMA* contained a full page ad for those imitation eggs."

Dr. Mary Enig and her associates at the University of Maryland published a series of papers severely damaging to the vegetable oil and margarine industries and the American government agencies urging a low-fat/cholesterol diet, specifically noting that the trans-fatty acids in such products produced dangerous changes in cells. One of the main findings Enig and her colleagues determined was that trans-fatty acids interfered with cellular enzyme systems that neutralized carcinogens, but increased enzymes that potentiated them, hence the high correlation between trans fat consumption and various cancers ("Modification of Membrane Lipid Composition..." 1984).

Enig became suspicious of the Lipid Hypothesis' validity when she realized that animal fat consumption had declined steadily since the turn of the century. For example, a report in the *Journal of American Oil Chemists* showed that animal fat consumption had declined from 104 grams per person per day in 1909, to 97 grams per day in 1972, while vegetable fat intake had increased from a low 21 grams to almost 60 grams. Total fat consumption had increased, as the proponents of the Lipid Hypothesis argued, but this increase was mostly due to vegetable oils with 50 percent coming from liquid oils and another 41 percent from margarine made from vegetable oils (Rizek, et. al. 244).

Enig and her colleagues wrote a detailed paper criticizing the Lipid Hypothesis' conclusion that there was a strong correlation between dietary saturated fat intake and the incidence of colon and breast cancer. The paper also demonstrated that the positive correlations between fat intake and cancer rates came from vegetable and trans fats, not the saturated fats of animals or coconuts. Indeed, Enig concluded that saturated fats seemed to *protect* against cancer! The paper was published in an American journal, *Federation Proceedings,* in July 1978 to the dismay of the vegetable oil industry. Enig and her colleagues lost all their funding money for research. The paper was subsequently viciously attacked by proponents of the Lipid Hypothesis and scientists employed by food companies, but Enig and her colleagues defended themselves well, at least in the scientific journals that printed their response letters; several journals refused to print her rebuttals to criticisms (Fallon & Enig "Oiling" 9-11).

Enig also began investigating the trans fat levels in a wide variety of foods on the market. Despite pressures from the food industry on the University to halt the research, Enig and her colleagues discovered disturbing things about the amount of trans fat consumption, as well as its effects on the body (mostly detailed in the next chapter).

Another well-known detractor was Dr. John Yudkin of Great Britain. In the 1950s, at the same time that Ancel Keys was promoting the Lipid Hypothesis, Yudkin and his colleagues published conclusive findings that excessive refined sugar intake was associated with elevated blood cholesterol, elevated triglycerides (blood fats), enlargement of the liver, increased corticosteroid levels in the blood, hypertrophy of the adrenal glands, and shrinkage of the pancreas (see all references for Yudkin in *Works Cited*). Other researchers, following Yudkin's lead, also looked into refined sugar's role in disease and discovered that ◆ *increased sugar intake was one of the main causes of heart disease* (Mudd). Yudkin's studies were ignored, too.

Dr. George Mann did independent studies on the Masai of East Africa (discussed below) that convinced him that the diet/heart hypothesis was a "scam." Calling the Lipid Hypothesis "the public health diversion of this century… the greatest scam in the history of medicine" (*Coronary Heart Disease* 1), Mann organized an "Anti-Lipid Hypothesis" conference, out of his own pocket of course, as the food industry and major government agencies refused to fund it. Mann invited several scientists and researchers, many of whom initially confirmed their attendance, and then backed out. Mann noted in his initial speech at the November 1991 conference, attended by a whopping seven participants, that:

> Scientists who must go before review panels for their research funding know well that to speak out, to disagree with this false dogma of Diet/Heart, is a fatal error. They must comply or go unfunded. I could show a list of scientists who said to me, in effect, when I invited them to participate, 'I believe you are right, that the Diet/Heart hypothesis is wrong, but I cannot join you because that would jeopardize my perks and funding.' For me, that kind of hypocritical response separates the scientists from the operators, the men from the boys (quoted in Fallon & Enig "Oiling" 9).

So, as is often the case in science, to dissent from the majority opinion is dangerous business, especially when research dollars are at stake. If you disagree, or if you show support or interest in those that do, you either lose your funding or are in danger of losing it. Other notable critics of the lipid hypothesis include Linus Pauling, PhD; Michael Gurr, PhD; Edward Pinckney, MD; Raymond Reiser, PhD; Russell Smith, PhD; and William Stehbens, MD.

It is time now to look at the evidence brought forward to support the Lipid Hypothesis, as well as the considerable evidence against it. It will be seen that the connection between diet and heart disease is not what most of you think.

THE VALIDITY OF THE LIPID HYPOTHESIS

The main points of the Lipid Hypothesis are as follows:

A. That saturated fat and cholesterol consumption has increased through the 20th century, with a corresponding increase in heart disease;

B. That dietary intake of cholesterol through cholesterol-containing foods raises blood cholesterol levels;

C. That increased blood cholesterol levels correlate with an increased risk and occurrence of CVD;

D. That saturated fats and cholesterol clog arteries in the form of arterial plaque;

E. That a high intake of saturated fat and cholesterol increases one's risk for CVD and that increased rates of CVD are seen in those who eat high fat/cholesterol diets;

F. That reducing one's intake of saturated fat and cholesterol, and increasing one's intake of unsaturated fats, translates to a decreased risk for CVD;

G. That numerous studies prove that increased dietary saturated fat/cholesterol intake strongly correlate with higher rates of atherosclerosis and heart disease.

Let's take a close look at each of these points.

THE POINTS ANALYZED

A. Saturated fat and cholesterol consumption has increased through the 20th century, with a corresponding increase in heart disease.

The quotations from Stamler and Ornish at the beginning of this chapter clearly stated this. Unfortunately, these claims are absolutely false. Anthropological data confirm that humans have always eaten meat and animal fat and, unless constrained by environmental or economical factors, preferred them as food sources over vegetable foods (Abrams, "Vegetarianism; The Preference for Animal Protein and Fat"). Paleolithic peoples apparently hunted certain species to extinction and the expansion of humanity across and around the globe was due to its quest for more animal foods (Abrams). Societies only turn to a diet of predominantly plant stuffs when absolutely necessary, and when they do, the effects are deleterious. For example, Abrams, citing Wells, notes that, "The dependence on high carbohydrate foods such as grain crops and other plant foods have resulted in undermining the health adaptations of food-producing populations unless they have been able to provide and maintain a balance between meat animals and their low protein crops" (Vegetarianism 73).

A cursory survey of dietary habits of native peoples from around the world flatly contradicts claims that humans ate less animal products than 20th century peoples. As noted in chapter two, all cultures show a preference for animal protein and animal fat and there is no such thing as a totally vegetarian culture anywhere in the world; veganism is primarily a 20th century phenomenon. For example, the Masai of East Africa, before modernization, consumed a diet of almost 100% animal products. The Eskimo, before they adopted civilized foods, also were almost 100% carnivorous. Australian Aborigines traditionally consume an array of animal products, including insects, supplemented by plant foods. And so forth and so on.

When it comes to Americans, and other Western peoples, a survey of any cookbook from the last century will quickly reveal what people were eating: lots of saturated fat from butter, cream, eggs, and lard (Fallon and Enig, "Americans…" 1-3). For example, the *Baptist Ladies Cookbook* (Monmouth, Illinois; 1895) contains recipes for such dishes as lamb croquettes, scalloped fish, creamed liver, creamed sweetbreads, creamed onions, and salmon with cheese sauce. An entire chapter of the cookbook is devoted to oysters with recipes such as oysters wrapped in bacon, scalloped oysters, and deviled oysters (made with eggs). A recipe for oyster pie calls for a quart of cream and a dozen egg yolks. The vegetable chapter reveals that creamed vegetable dishes were quite popular. There are recipes for creamed cabbage, creamed cucumbers, and parsnips fried in bacon fat, among many others. Even sugary desserts contained substantial amounts of saturated fats. A recipe for German waffles, for example, calls for an entire pound of butter and 12 eggs.

Recipes from the *Boston Cooking School Cookbook* (Boston, Massachusetts; 1896) are similar to those of the Baptists with meal suggestions that go like this:

Breakfast: Oatmeal with sugar and cream; creamed fish; baked potatoes; corncakes; coffee with cream

Lunch: Lamb croquettes fried in lard; "dressed" lettuce; biscuits with butter; gingerbread; cheese

Dinner: Soup with cream or whole milk; meat or fish with scalloped potatoes; two other vegetable dishes, usually creamed; vegetable salad; crackers, cheese, and coffee with cream

A caloric analysis of some of these menus reveals up to 40% of calories coming from fat, with a slightly higher ratio of saturated to unsaturated fats (Fallon and Enig "Americans" 3). Recipes from a Jewish housewives cookbook published in London, England, in 1846 reveal similar recipes with tallow being substituted for lard.

The *Searchlight Recipe Book* (1931), also has similar recipes for creamed fish and organ meats, along with dessert recipes with lots of butter and eggs, and vegetable dishes with a cream or cheese sauce. One thing very noticeable in this later cookbook, however, is the option in some recipes of using butter or a "butter substitute," i.e., margarine. Some recipes also call for "vegetable oil." This cookbook clearly shows the substitution of vegetable fats for animal fats. Only a few years later, heart disease was pandemic.

On a more scientific level, food data from the United States Department of Agriculture (USDA) shows that animal fat consumption, especially of butter, has steadily declined in this century, but that vegetable oil and margarine consumption, i.e., polyunsaturated fats, has gone up tremendously (*USDA- HNI; ENIG* 89-112). A report published in the *Journal of the American Oil Chemist's Society* demonstrated that animal fat consumption was substantially higher at the beginning of this century compared to now (Rizek 244).

While it is true that meat consumption has risen in the last few decades, the rise has mostly been from increased chicken consumption, specifically recommended by the Prudent Diet. Chicken, however, is low in saturated fat. Even chicken skin, recommended not to be eaten, contains appreciable amounts of PUFA's. Beef and pork consumption, the highly saturated fat meats, has risen as well and some try to use these data to prove that animal food/fat intake therefore correlates with higher CVD rates, but it is not mentioned that intake of margarine, trans-fats, refined sugar, and processed foods has also risen, quite astronomically in fact. Laying the blame on meat products and saturated fat, while ignoring these other factors, is very bad reasoning indeed.

The first claim, then, of the Lipid Hypothesis cannot be supported by any factual data. If anything, the data supports the **opposite** of the Lipid Hypothesis: ◆ *as animal fat consumption has decreased and vegetable fat consumption has increased, heart disease and cancer have increased!*

B. Dietary intake of cholesterol through cholesterol-containing foods raises blood cholesterol levels.

It is claimed by supporters of the Lipid Hypothesis that cholesterol-rich foods like whole milk, cheese, meat, eggs, liver, and shellfish raise blood cholesterol levels when eaten. There is a mountain of evidence to demonstrate that this is not true.

When Dr. George Mann of Vanderbilt University studied the Masai, a people whose diet mostly consists of beef, whole milk, and blood, he found they had serum cholesterol levels well within the "normal" range. He also discovered that they had very little, if any, CVD.

A study conducted by Hitchcock and Bracey in Busselton, Australia, studied three groups of mothers and children; one with high cholesterol, one with medium, and one with low cholesterol levels. They studied diet patterns of each group and found there was no significant difference among their daily food intakes. In other words, their diet had no bearing on their cholesterol levels (35).

A group of New Guinea natives whose diets were very low in cholesterol were given eggs in an experiment designed to measure how the eggs would affect cholesterol levels. Their cholesterol levels remained the same; the eggs had no effect on their cholesterol levels (NEJM 98:317-323, 1978).

◆ *Studies conducted on diet and cholesterol levels by other researchers found no significant difference in plasma cholesterol levels in egg eaters and non-egg eaters* (Reiser, 22-28; Slater, et al, 249; Porter, et al, 490).

The liver manufactures most of the cholesterol it needs for an assortment of biochemical processes, about 2 grams a day. Only about 100 mg is absorbed from food in the small intestines, a tiny amount to be sure, but this quantity is needed by the body to give it the substrates necessary to manufacture enough (Fallon and Enig "Oiling" 11). Eliminating cholesterol foods from one's diet, then, is ill advised.

Indeed, Dr. Enig accurately points out in her book, *Know Your Fats*, that "in fact there is evidence that for some people cholesterol is an absolute dietary essential because their own synthesis is not adequate." And further that, "the effect of natural fatty acids on serum cholesterol levels is dependent on the original serum cholesterol levels: high serum cholesterol *decreases* with consumption of most fatty acids, including all saturates; low serum cholesterol *increases* with many of the fatty acids, including saturates, monounsaturates, and sometimes polyunsaturates" (57). In other words, if your cholesterol level is too high for your individual needs, eating saturated fats will help lower and normalize it. If, however, your level is too low for your needs, eating fatty acids of all types will help raise and normalize it.

C. Increased blood cholesterol levels correlate with an increased risk and occurrence of CVD.

Despite what the public, and supporters of the Lipid Hypothesis, think, ◆ *most people, over 80%, do NOT have elevated cholesterol levels prior to experiencing a heart attack* (Rowland, 18; Ravnskov 47-93). Abrams concurs: "There is no positive or direct proof that high cholesterol levels results in heart disease ("Vegetarianism 63). Dr. Michael DeBakey, the world renowned heart surgeon from Houston, has done extensive research into the Lipid Hypothesis, specifically the dietary cholesterol aspect. He found that only 30 or 40% of people with atherosclerosis or CVD actually have elevated cholesterol levels. He stated: "If you say cholesterol is the cause, how do you explain the other 60% to 70% with heart disease who don't have high cholesterol?" (Reiser 22-28). DeBakey made an analysis of 1,700 patients with CVD from hospital records. He found there was no definitive relationship or correlation between serum cholesterol and the extent of CVD (655-659). Reiser cites a study in which men from Crete and Crevalcore, Italy, with similar cholesterol levels, nevertheless had different rates of CVD.

It would appear, then, that serum cholesterol is not an indicator of either heart disease or risk of it. There are, however, small numbers of people who possess a genetic defect that interferes with their body's ability to metabolize cholesterol. This condition is called "hypercholesterolemia." These people DO have to watch their blood cholesterol levels. As Dr. Uffe Ravnskov points out in his excellent book, *The Cholesterol Myths*, most of the studies done demonstrating positive correlations between cholesterol levels and heart disease have been performed on people with this condition, but one cannot apply data from a group of people with a metabolic defect to the general population who do not share the same problem.

D. Saturated fats and cholesterol clog arteries in the form of arterial plaque.

The rabbit studies done by Kritchevsky are offered as proof that this point is true. Unfortunately, the basis of the experiment is flawed: rabbits are herbivorous creatures, therefore, they lack the physiological traits required to assimilate and metabolize cholesterol which is only found in animal products. It is no wonder, then, that Kritchevsky's rabbits developed problems. One cannot apply the results of an experiment done on herbivores to an omnivorous species like humans (Rowland 19).

A study in the medical journal *Lancet* (1994, 344:1195) demonstrated that the fatty acids in arterial plaque are mostly *unsaturated* (74%), of which **41%** are polyunsaturated. This finding flatly contradicts the Lipid Hypothesis. It is consistent, however, with what we know about excessive PUFAs, they are bad news. The studies that Kritchevsky did with his rabbits were actually done with powdered cholesterol mixed with corn oil, a predominantly PUFA (Fallon and Enig, "Oiling," 12).

The evidence for saturated fat clogging arteries is so flimsy that eminent biochemist, Dr. Michael Gurr, stated in a recent article, "Whatever is the cause of heart disease, it is not primarily the consumption of saturated fats." Gurr then went on to criticize "the degree of self delusion in research workers wedded to a particular hypothesis despite the contrary evidence!" (432-435).

As Rowland points out (18-20), cholesterol is a slippery, waxy substance that moves at a high rate of speed. It is, therefore, impossible that it could "stick" to arterial walls which are very smooth. He also points out that, "There is just as much cholesterol in our veins as in our arteries; but plaque is always found only in arteries and never in veins. If cholesterol were the cause of circulatory disease, then surely it would damage veins as much as arteries. But it does not."

Then why is cholesterol found in arterial plaque? Because the arteries have been damaged by something else and the body uses cholesterol as a repair substance (Cranton and Frackelton 6-37). Furthermore, cholesterol is one of the last substances to be laid down in arterial plaque, not the first (Rowland 18). It is, therefore, impossible that it could be the cause of arterial clogs.

What is the cause? In answering this question, one must realize first that all peoples, no matter what their diet, experience some atherosclerosis; it is a consequence of aging. The 1968 International Atherosclerosis Project, in which over 22,000 corpses in 14 countries were autopsied for arterial plaque, showed arterial degeneration in all subjects—in populations that suffered from a great deal of heart disease, and in populations that did not (McGill, et al. 498). What the difference is, though, is the degree of blockage. Having a fatty-streaked artery is quite different from having a totally occluded one. As we shall see in the following chapter, the primary culprits in arterial clogs are processed vegetable oils, refined sugars, assorted nutritional deficiencies and oxidized cholesterol (the kind used by Kritchevsky in his experiments).

E. A high intake of saturated fat and cholesterol increases one's risk for CVD and that increased rates of CVD are seen in those who eat high fat/cholesterol diets.

As we learned in our study of Dr. Price's work, ◆ *native peoples the world over consume high amounts of animal fats with little incidence of heart disease.* For example, the Masai and related tribes of East Africa subsist largely on beef, whole milk, and blood. Yemenite Jews eat a diet containing fats solely of animal origin, yet have an almost zero incidence of heart disease and hypertension. Peoples living in northern India consume 17 times more animal fat than people living in southern India, but have an incidence of CVD seven times LOWER than in southern India. Eskimos eat liberally of animal fats, both from fish and marine mammals, yet, as long as they stay on their native diet, enjoy freedom from CVD, obesity, osteoporosis, diabetes, and cancer. Several Mediterranean societies are free of CVD, even though fat consumption accounts for up to 70% of their diet. A study of Puerto Ricans revealed that, in spite of a high animal fat intake, they have low rates of colon and breast cancer (studies summarized in Fallon, Enig, and Connolly 7; see also Ravnskov 32-46).

Ancel Keys claimed that the Japanese had the lowest incidence of CVD because of their low fat diet in his Seven Countries study, but this is not altogether true. The Japanese consume moderate amounts of fat and substantial amounts of cholesterol from their diet of seafoods and shellfish. Additionally, the Swiss, the second longest living people in the world right behind the Japanese, eat a diet loaded with saturated fat from dairy products.

Most of us have heard of the "French Paradox." It refers to the fact that although the typical French diet is loaded with eggs, cream, butter, cheeses, and rich pates, the French people have a much lower incidence of CVD than people in the United States. Some researchers, not willing to let the Lipid Hypothesis go in the face of this embarrassing evidence, claim the French are protected from all of their dietary saturated fat and cholesterol by the antioxidants in red wine, which the French drink.

Unfortunately, not every French person drinks wine; I know because I've lived in France! Furthermore, high cholesterol levels, high saturated fat intake and low heart disease rates exist in countries like Germany and Luxemborg where red wine is not part of the daily diet (Ravnskov 72). While there may be antioxidant benefits in grapes, it is unlikely that they are protecting the French from CVD.

With all of this contrary evidence, how could anyone possibly hold the Lipid Hypothesis to be true? The problem is that researchers fail to properly isolate specific dietary factors in their subjects. We saw this at the beginning of this chapter: Garrison and Somer lumped together ice cream and margarine right along with butter and beef. Yet any person with common sense knows that these foods are not identical. The fats in these foods are also vastly different.

◆ *Modern researchers fail to properly isolate dietary factors in people with CVD or cancer.* As a result, the harmful effects of trans fat (and sugar) consumption (discussed fully in the next chapter), get mixed up with SFA consumption (Byrnes, "Facing the Facts…" 33). The result is that SFAs get blamed for the evils of trans fats, excessive PUFAs, and refined sugars. This is actually how the Lipid Hypothesis got its start: in the 1940s, American researchers found a strong correlation between cancer and fat consumption—the fats used were hydrogenated fats, not naturally saturated fats (Enig, *Nutrition Quarterly*). The error has been repeated ever since despite a number of studies clearly exonerating animal fats as causes of either heart disease or cancer. A good example of this is the result of a long term study of 60,000 Scandinavian women reported in the *Archives of Internal Medicine*. The authors noted that animal fat consumption, even when high, did not translate into an increased risk for cancer, unlike vegetable oils and other polyunsaturates (Wolk, et al.). Other US studies, such as the Veterans Clinical Trial, the Minnesota State Hospital Trial, the Honolulu Heart Program, and the Puerto Rico Heart Health Study, found no correlation between a diet high in saturated fats and cholesterol with CVD (Fallon and Enig "Diet and Heart Disease" 2)

Rowland, lamenting the sad state of exacting research among supporters of the Lipid Hypothesis, stated: "I believe many of the ill effects attributed to eating meat [and fat] are misplaced. Western diets that are high in meat also tend to be low in dietary fibre and high in refined sugar and adulterated fats. Is it only one dietary culprit that is to blame or the combination of all?" ("As I See It" 3)

F. Reducing one's intake of saturated fat and cholesterol, and increasing one's intake of unsaturated fats, translates to a decreased risk for CVD.

Since we have already seen that dietary cholesterol has little effect on serum cholesterol levels, and that a high intake of SFAs does not correlate with greater risk for cancer or heart disease (remember, here, how study results get confused because of poor dietary analyses), the first part of this contention is wrong. The second, however, deserves our attention.

Kritchevsky's studies did show that PUFAs reduced serum cholesterol levels. The likely explanation for this is that as PUFAs are increasingly incorporated into our cell membranes, they become weaker. The body then sequesters cholesterol from the blood to add "stiffness" to the cellular membrane (Fallon and Enig, "Oiling," 15). The result is a reduction of serum cholesterol levels. But remember: there is no proof that such a reduction translates into a reduction of risk for CVD.

While small amounts of PUFAs are needed by the body, their excessive consumption is extremely deleterious to the body (discussed fully in the next chapter). How tragic that, for the past 50 years, Westerners have been urged to consume more PUFAs in the form of vegetable oils. This advice has translated into nothing but death and suffering.

Finally, early in 1998 a symposium entitled "Evolution of Ideas about the Nutritional Value of Dietary Fat" reviewed the flaws of the Lipid Hypothesis, as well as studies that showed that mice fed whole milk lived several months longer than mice on fat-free milk. One of the participants noted that low fat diets and cholesterol-lowering drugs in study trials "did not affect overall CHD [coronary heart disease] mortality." This person also went on to say, "Research continues apace and, as new findings appear, it may be necessary to re-evaluate our conclusions and preventive medicine policies" (Olson, 421-425). Who made such statements? David Kritchevsky, the father of the Lipid Hypothesis!

G. Numerous studies prove that increased dietary saturated fat/cholesterol intake strongly correlates with higher rates of atherosclerosis and heart disease.

There have been a number of studies completed that supposedly prove the Lipid Hypothesis of heart disease. As we shall see from the following analysis, these studies actually prove little and, in fact, present data that confounds the Lipid Hypothesis. Let us go through the major studies one by one.

44

1. The Framingham Heart Study is often brought up to prove the Lipid Hypothesis. This study began in 1948 and involved about 6,000 people from a small town in Massachusetts. Two groups were compared at five year intervals—one group ate lots of saturated fat and cholesterol, and another group ate little. One major finding of the study was that those who weighed more and had higher blood cholesterol levels were more at risk for CVD. Weight gain and cholesterol levels, however, had an INVERSE correlation with dietary intake of fat and cholesterol. In other words, there was no correlation whatsoever. Dr. William Castelli, MD, headed the study and had to admit in 1992:

   > In Framingham, Massachusetts, the more saturated fat one ate, the more cholesterol one ate, the more calories one ate, the lower people's serum cholesterol…we found that the people who ate the most cholesterol, ate the most saturated fat, ate the most calories, weighed the least and were the most physically active (Castelli, 1371-1372).

2. In a multi-year British study involving several thousand men, half were asked to reduce saturated fat and cholesterol, to stop smoking, and to increase their intakes of margarine and vegetable oils. After a year, those on the "good" diet had 100% more deaths than those on the "bad" one, even though these men continued to smoke! In describing the study, however, the lead researcher ignored these results and urged that the British public follow the "good" diet designed by the study's authors (Rose, et al, 1062-1065).

3. The US Multiple Risk Factor Intervention Trial compared mortality rates and eating habits of 12,000+ men. Those with "good" dietary habits, i.e., low saturated fat, reduced smoking, etc., showed a **slight** reduction in total CVD rates, but their all cause death rate was higher than the "bad" group. This result has been repeated many times in other similar studies, but it is never revealed to the public. The few studies that indicate a correlation between fat reduction and a decrease in CVD mortality also clearly document a sizeable increase in deaths from cancer, suicide, and violence (*JAMA*, 1982, 1465).

4. The Lipid Research Clinics Coronary Primary Prevention Trial is, like the Framingham study, always brought forward to support the

Lipid Hypothesis. But this study did not actually test for dietary cholesterol and saturated fat intake as all the subjects involved were already on a low fat diet. Instead, the study tested the effects of a cholesterol-lowering drug. Statistical analysis of the results indicated a 24% reduction in the rate of CVD in the drug-taking group compared to the other who took no drug at all. Deaths, however, from cancer, stroke, violence, and suicide rose considerably in the drug-taking group. The 24% reduction claim was challenged later by independent researchers. They found NO statistical difference in the CVD rates between both groups. Despite these disturbing data, the press and medical communities hailed the Trial as proof that animal fats killed people and that lowering cholesterol was good (*JAMA*, 1984, 359; Kronmal, 2091).

5. Another popular study was the Leiden Intervention Trial conducted in the Netherlands. Over 10 years ago, the elderly people of this small town had their cholesterol levels measured and were placed on a low cholesterol/saturated fat diet. A decade later, investigators made the shocking discovery that those who had higher serum cholesterol levels lived longer than those with lower levels. Those with a cholesterol level of 251+ had a 44% lower mortality rate than those whose readings were 194 or less (*Lancet*, 1997, 11). So much for longevity and low cholesterol levels.

6. Even Keys' famous "Seven Countries Study," thought to establish the Lipid Hypothesis by showing that high rates of CVD correlated with high intakes of saturated fat ("Diet and Development…"), was severely flawed:

> His evidence for contending that animal fat causes heart disease was based on two kinds of data: a comparison of widely different groups' cause of death as listed on death certificates and data on the diet of the nation [not the individual] and the level of serum cholesterol. From these rather unreliable types of data, he concluded a high intake of animal fats causes a high level of serum cholesterol which in turn leads to coronary heart disease (Abrams "Vegetarianism" 69).

Keys claimed that the country with the highest animal fat intake and the highest cholesterol levels (at that time, Finland) had the highest heart disease rates, while the country with the lowest (at that time, Japan) had the lowest. Keys claimed there was a cause and effect relationship. Most people, however, do not know that Keys *hand-picked* the countries to include in his famous study, namely, the ones that fit into his hypothesis about heart disease. Keys conveniently ignored all the other countries that had high saturated fat intakes and high cholesterol levels, but had *low* heart disease rates (for example, France and Sweden at that time—see Ravnskov 75-77).

Yudkin also demonstrated that Keys ignored refined sugar intakes of his study subjects. Yudkin determined that in the same countries that Keys studied in a 1953 paper, the correlation between refined sugar intake and CVD was much higher than that between fat and CVD. Yudkin specifically criticised Keys saying, "No one has ever shown any difference in fat consumption between people with and people without coronary diseases, but this has in no way deterred Dr. Keys and his followers" (quoted in Pauling, 53).

7. Dean Ornish, MD, is a popular American doctor who claimed to have statistically proved that a low fat, low cholesterol diet could reverse and prevent CVD. "The Ornish Plan" is well-known and heavily advocated for CVD. Unfortunately, it appears that the dietary component of Ornish's plan has little effect on CVD. Ornish not only takes a dietary approach to CVD, but also encourages life-style changes such as daily meditation, stress reduction exercises, exercise, and smoking cessation. In a recent advertisement for Ornish's products, it was revealed that:

> For the first time, 'Dr. Ornish's research offers strong scientific evidence that life-style changes *alone* [emphasis added] can actually begin to reverse even severe coronary artery disease after only one year without the use of cholesterol-lowering drugs' (Claude Lenfant, M.D., Director, National heart, Lung, and Blood Institute, National Institutes of Health). Patients reported a 91% reduction in the frequency of chest pains, and for most of them, the progression of arterial clogging reversed after only one year. In contrast, heart disease *worsened* for the majority of patients in the control group, *who exercised moderately and followed a conventional 'low fat' diet* [emphasis added].

In commenting on Ornish's studies, Dr. Russell Smith wrote "the amount of [arterial] regression did not correlate with the amount of cholesterol reduction. This was a most significant finding that was not discussed in Ornish's paper when all subjects had completed the 1-year program" (6-38). Dr. Smith, Ph.D., authored a massive analysis of all studies done that supposedly prove the Lipid Hypothesis and showed in painstaking detail how study results were manipulated to prove the theory. In one revealing section of his book, he shows that, in some study groups, death rates *decreased* as people consumed *more* saturated fat and cholesterol! Smith also constantly points out how all studies showing the Lipid Hypothesis to be true are sponsored, either all or in part, by various companies who manufacture cholesterol-lowering drugs, or who make low fat foods. The validity of these studies is, of course, very suspect given the sponsors. If you are so inclined, I urge you to acquire a copy.

A dietary approach to CVD and hypertension that does not receive much attention from the medical world is the program of popular diet writer Dr. Robert Atkins, MD, of New York. Atkins treats his CVD patients with a high protein, high fat, high cholesterol, but low carbohydrate, diet with much success. Such clinical evidence is an embarrassment to the Lipid Hypothesis, but it demonstrates the point of this chapter: saturated fat and cholesterol do not cause heart disease.

HDL-LDL

A number of studies seem to indicate that low levels of High Density Lipoproteins (HDL) and high levels of Low Density Lipoproteins (LDL) translate into an increased risk for heart disease. HDL is often referred to as the "good cholesterol," and LDL as the "bad" one. Some studies show that a reduction of saturated fat intake raises HDL levels (but others show the opposite—see references to Dr. Mary Enig's work in the bibliography). In short, HDL's carry cholesterol in the blood back to the liver for breakdown, while LDL's carry cholesterol from the liver out to tissues (Garrison and Somer 348). It is routine for people to have their ratios of HDL to LDL checked when going for a medical exam or blood work.

It appears, however, that the HDL-LDL theory is unfounded. Smith cites numerous studies where there was no significant relationship between HDL or LDL levels and heart disease (vol 2:1-1 to 1-5; 3-78 to

3-102). He quotes Lipid Hypothesis supporters Grundy, Rifkin, and Cleeman as saying:

> Often, populations with a high prevalence of CHD have relatively HIGH [emphasis added] HDL concentrations… Moreover, there are populations… in which low HDL cholesterol concentrations seemingly do not convey increased risk for CHD. Finally, certain genetic causes of severely **reduced** HDL apparently **are not accompanied by a markedly increased coronary risk** [emphasis added] (3-89).

Smith then cites research from Knuiman, et al, demonstrating that, among different populations from different countries, there is no significant relationship between HDL levels and heart disease (3-89). Smith also cites research from Lewis, et al, who reported that HDL levels were almost identical in large samples of men and women from Italy, Switzerland, England, and Sweden, but that deaths from heart disease differed among these countries (3-89-90). If the HDL-LDL theory were true, then there should have been a consistent death rate from heart disease since all of the subjects had similar HDL levels, but such was not the case.

ONE LIPOPROTEIN TO WORRY ABOUT

Is **lipoprotein** (a). Even the conservative Garrison and Somer warn against Lp(a): "Evidence implicates elevated levels of Lp(a) as an independent risk factor for CVD. Some researchers suggest that Lp(a) promotes atherosclerosis …." (349) Dr. Joseph Mercola, an osteopath, writes in his online newsletter, "Elevated lipoprotein A levels are a serious risk factor for cardiovascular disease. We screen all of our chelation patients for this" (11). Dr. Mary Enig describes Lp(a) as "atherogenic" ("Fat Facts," 14). Though research is still continuing on this substance, ◆ *it is recommended that you request your Lp(a) levels be measured at your next checkup.* Acceptable levels per dl of blood would be <10 mg. 11-24 md/dl are borderline high; >25 are very high. If your Lp (a) levels are over 10, you need to take action at once.

What raises Lp(a) levels? Trans-fatty acids. What lowers them? Saturated fats! (Enig, "Fat Facts," 14) Mercola states that he uses a combination of vitamin C, niacin, and the amino acids lysine and proline to lower Lp(a) levels. This is similar to the protocol advocated by Dr. Mathias Rath, former research colleague of Dr. Linus Pauling.

SATURATED FATS: WHAT YOU HAVEN'T BEEN TOLD

Many people, because of the anti-fat propaganda of the last 50 years, think there is nothing nutritious about saturated fats, but there are many vital nutrients and substances found in saturated fats not found in other foods. Butter, for example, is rich in trace minerals, particularly selenium, all the fat-soluble vitamins, as well as two fatty acids: butyric and lauric. Both of these are antifungal, antibacterial, and antineoplastic (against cancer) substances. Additionally, butter provides the fatty material needed by the intestines to convert plant carotenes into active vitamin A. Due to the unjustified saturated fat and cholesterol scare of the past few decades, most people have eliminated butter from their diets. These people would probably reconsider this decision if they knew of butter's healthful qualities but health authorities never relate them.

Coconut oil is another good example. Formerly used widely in baked goods, this oil is very rich in lauric acid. This fatty acid converts in the intestines into *monolaurin*, a powerful antifungal and antibacterial substance. Coconut oil also contains caprylic acid, also a powerful antifungal. Yet these properties are lost amidst a plethora of unwarranted warnings about "the dangers of saturated fat." Tropical peoples have had coconut as an integral part of their diet for thousands of years, yet suffer from no CVD, as long as they remain on their native diet.

The body needs saturated fats in order to properly utilize essential fatty acids. Saturated fats also lower the blood levels of the artery-damaging lipoprotein (a), elevate HDL levels, are needed for proper calcium utilization in the bones, and provide a good energy source for the vital organs. They stimulate the immune system, protect the liver, do not initiate free radical formation, and are non-irritating to the arterial walls. Omitting them from one's diet, then, is poor advice indeed! (Kabara, 1-14; Watkins, et al., "Importance of Vitamin E..."; Watkins and Seifert, 101; Mead, et al, *Lipids*; Nanji, et al, 547-554; Cha and Sachan, 338-343; Garg, et al, A852; Oliart Ros, at al, 7).

THE DANGERS OF THE PRUDENT DIET

You should have noticed that ◆ *subjects placed on low fat/cholesterol diets and given cholesterol-lowering drugs suffered from serious health problems.* This is not difficult to understand. Cholesterol is needed by the body to manufacture an array of hormones, as well as contribute to the structural integrity of the cell wall. Cholesterol is also needed for the proper function of serotonin receptors in the brain. Serotonin is what makes us "feel" good; this is why low cholesterol levels are associated with higher rates of depression, suicide, and aggressive behavior. Dietary cholesterol plays an important role in maintaining the health of the intestinal wall. People on low cholesterol diets tend to suffer from gastrointestinal problems, including "Leaky Gut Syndrome." As a practitioner who has dealt with several former "low fat folk," I can clinically attest to this. Cholesterol is also needed for the proper development of the brain and nervous system. This is one of the reasons why human breast milk contains high amounts of saturated fat and cholesterol. Despite this, and the fact that low fat diets cause learning disabilities, stunted growth, and failure to thrive, major public health organizations recommend low fat/cholesterol diets for children! One can only lament the fate of these unfortunate innocents (references for this section are summarized and listed by Fallon and Enig, "Oiling," 11-12; see also Ravnskov 230-231).

Since fat provides a reliable energy source to the body, ◆*low fat diets are associated with depression, low energy, and fatigue.* Additionally, since saturated animal fats are carriers of the fat-soluble vitamins (A, D, E, and K), and since the body needs such nutrients to properly assimilate protein, omitting them from one's diet is ill-advised. Remember Dr. Price's research: diets of robust primitives contained 10 times the amount of fat-soluble vitamins than modern diets at that time.

Some people have reservations about adding more butter, cream, and coconut into their diets for they fear they will gain weight from consuming more fat. This is not altogether true. The fatty acids the body stores as fat tissue are the long and very long ones, the kind found more in olive and vegetable oils; the short and medium length ones are used for energy and not stored. About 15% of the fatty acids in butter and about 65% of the fatty acids in coconut are of the short and medium chain variety—weight gain is unlikely.

As we leave this chapter and move on to the real and varied causes of heart disease, remember two things: (1) animal fats like butter and cream really are good for you and do not contribute to CVD, and (2) vegetable oils and margarine are not and do—don't buy or consume them in the future.

KEY POINTS TO REMEMBER

> ◆ *Dr. Price's studies of real people and what they actually ate show that a high intake of saturated fat produced robust health.*

◆ *The more a fat is saturated, the more stable it is chemically.*

◆ *It is mostly trans-fatty acid consumption and not saturated fat consumption that is strongly correlated with increased cancer and cardiovascular disease.*

◆ *In times when heart disease and MI's were rare, people consumed plenty of animal fats, namely, butter, lard, cream, eggs, and tallow.*

◆ *Increased sugar intake is one of the main causes of heart disease.*

◆ *As animal fat consumption has decreased and vegetable fat consumption has increased, heart disease and cancer have increased.*

◆ *Studies conducted on diet and cholesterol levels found no significant difference in plasma cholesterol levels in egg eaters and non-egg eaters.*

◆ *Most people do NOT have elevated cholesterol levels prior to experiencing a heart attack.*

◆ *Native peoples the world over consume high amounts of animal fats with no incidence of heart disease.*

◆ *Modern researchers fail to properly isolate dietary factors in people with CVD or cancer.*

◆ *It is recommended that you request your Lp(a) levels be measured at your next checkup.*

◆ *Subjects placed on low fat/cholesterol diets and who took cholesterol-lowering drugs suffered from serious health problems.*

◆ *Low fat diets are associated with depression, low energy, and fatigue.*

CHAPTER FOUR

The Real
Villains

Now that we know that saturated fat and cholesterol doesn't cause heart disease, what does? As I said at the beginning of this book, heart disease is a multifaceted disease with several causes contributing to it. In this chapter, we'll take a look at most of them. Basically, one can divide the assorted causes for CVD into three groups: Dietary Dangers, Nutritional Deficiencies, and Life-style Factors.

DIETARY DANGERS

1. REFINED SUGARS

We mentioned the work of Dr. John Yudkin of Great Britain in the last chapter. Yudkin showed that increased refined sugar consumption caused a host of health problems, including accelerated atherosclerosis and heart disease. In 1957, Yudkin reported a study from the death rate of CVD in fifteen countries in relation to the average intake of sugar. The annual death rate from CVD per 100,000 persons increases steadily from 60 for an intake of 20 pounds of sugar per year to 300 for 120 pounds per year, and then 750 for 150 pounds per year (Pauling, 53). This is extremely damning evidence to refined sugars. ◆ *Wherever refined sugar goes, dental decay and disease follow.*

We need to define what refined sugar is a little more so we can better understand why it is so harmful. The energy of food is contained in proteins, fats, and carbohydrates. Carbs are broken down into two groups: simple and complex. Complex carbs are found in whole grains, legumes, seeds, and starchy vegetables. They, generally, take longer to digest than their relatives, the simple carbs. Simple carbs are your simple sugars, glucose, fructose, lactose, etc. Refined grain products also qualify as simple sugars. Simple carbs are broken down into two types as well: natural and refined.

What's the difference between a natural, simple carb and a refined one? Naturally sweet foods like fruit, maple syrup, honey, corn, sugar cane and beets are linked together with the vitamins, minerals, and enzymes needed for their digestion and assimilation by the body. In measured amounts, all of these foods are healthful. But when the sugars in these foods are removed by refining, the sugars now exist SEPARATE from the nutrients. These "skeletonized" sugars are harmful to you. They are empty, negative calories that sap the body's nutrient reserves. The refining process also strips whole grains of both their B vitamin and mineral content.

While our ancestors ate some natural simple sugars (honey, maple syrup, sugar cane, fruits), **refined** simple sugars are new additions to the human diet—we did not evolve eating them. Since we did not evolve eating them, our bodies are not equipped to handle them. Refined sugars, therefore, do not belong in our diets. 100 years ago, sugar consumption was perhaps 12 lbs per person a year. Today, it is up to about 170 (Fallon, Enig, and Connolly, 21). That, combined with excessive amounts of polyunsaturated oils, makes a potent recipe for disease.

Studies have also shown that a high simple sugar intake depresses your immune system. When large amounts of simple sugars are eaten, your white blood cells are literally "stunned" for several hours, and unable to do their job of defending your body against invading microbes. And there's even more.

As early as 1933, research showed that increased sugar consumption caused an increase in various diseases in school children. Sugar has been shown to shorten the life span of lab animals. Some researchers blame refined sugar consumption as the root cause of anorexia and other eating disorders. Excessive sugar consumption has been conclusively linked to high blood cholesterol, liver enlargement, shrinkage of the adrenal glands and pancreas, candidiasis, heart disease, kidney disease, hyperactivity, behavior problems, poor concentration, violent tendencies, cancer (cancer cells are enormous sugar consumers), bone loss, obesity, and tooth decay (Fallon, Enig, and Connolly, 21-22; Abrams, "Hominid Proclivity for Sweetness," 35-42; Hoffer, 88-90; Pauling, 363).

Researchers who have followed Yudkin's lead have confirmed over and over that refined carbohydrates, such as processed sugar, white flour, and white rice, are deleterious to our health, especially our circulatory systems and hearts (Cleave; Steffanson; Page; Burkitt; Price; Hess; Williams).

One of the consequences of a high sugar intake is a higher insulin level; this, and insulin resistance, has been positively correlated with a proneness to heart disease (DeFronzo and Ferrannini; Zavoroni, et al; Reaven; Atkins).

More recent research has indicated that excess sugar in the bloodstream stimulates the generation of tissue-damaging and mutagenic substances called free radicals (discussed later in this chapter) and simultaneously lowers blood levels of vitamin E, a ptetent antioxidant very key in preventing heart disease and cancer (*Jnl of Clin Endocrin & Metab*, August 2000).

It is true that certain groups of people have consumed refined carbohydrates for a long time, with a low incidence of CVD, the British, for example. Although their teeth suffered, their overall health was fairly good. The likely explanation for this is in the overall high quality of the rest of their diet which included organ meats, healthy fats, and nutrient-dense grains and vegetables (Fallon and Enig, "Merrie Olde England;" "Americans, Then and Now").

The next step you need to take should be obvious: Throw out any refined sugar in your home. Avoid buying foods with a high sugar content (check all labels). In short, learn to live without refined sugar. Your heart and body will thank you for it.

Some of you may be tempted to use sugar substitutes to avoid the dangers of refined sucrose, but this is not really a good idea as numerous harmful side effects have been attributed to aspartame (including heart palpitations) and saccharin. It is far better wean yourself of your sweet tooth and to use natural sugars like maple syrup, raw honey (do not give to babies), sucanat, and black strap molasses in moderation. In most countries stevia, a South American herb, is available. It is an excellent, non-caloric sweetening agent.

2. POLYUNSATURATED OILS

Westerners have increasingly consumed more vegetable oils in this century and CVD rates have skyrocketed. Though other factors, especially refined sugar consumption, have contributed to this, the increasing ingestion of PUFAs is the major cause.

In the last chapter we noted that PUFAs, because of their chemical structure, are more fragile chemically; they break down and go rancid more easily than either MUFAs or SFAs. When oils go rancid, they give rise to substances called free radicals. These are unstable, tissue-damaging, and carcinogenic compounds that attack cellular membranes and alter DNA. Free radicals like attacking PUFAs, present in arterial walls, which leads to tears. The body attempts to repair the damage by sending calcium and cholesterol to the damage site. These solidify and arterial plaque begins to form.

Virtually all commercial vegetable oils, even those labeled "cold pressed," are rancid when purchased. Usually rancid oils smell, but manufacturers deodorize the oil before releasing it to stores, so you don't notice anything wrong. The reason why the oils are rancid is because of the high heat and pressure used to extract them from their original foods like corn, soybeans, or cottonseed. ♦ *Heat, light, and oxygen damage oils and denature them, eventually turning them rancid.*

But there are other dangers of PUFAs, besides their artery-damaging properties. Nutritional anthropologist H. Leon Abrams, Jr., explains:

> Studies strongly indicate that large consumptions of margarines, and other polyunsaturated vegetable fats may be conducive to cancer. Animal experiments found that rats fed a chemical carcinogen in addition to 20% vegetable polyunsaturated fat had a much higher incidence of tumors than when fed a carcinogen with animal fat. In a similar experiment, rats treated with a carcinogen and given 5% corn oil had a 3.5 times higher incidence of colon tumors than did rats who were maintained on 5% lard. Studies have also linked a high intake of polyunsaturates... with vitamin deficiencies, liver damage, premature aging, nutritional muscular dystrophy, cancer, and severe blood diseases in infants. Polyunsaturated fatty acids are believed to be highly reactive chemical compounds that render them possibly harmful; they can be oxidized by ordinary cooking, in one's body when they react with nitrous oxide in smog, from X-rays and sunlight and some trace metals such as iron. ("Vegetarianism," 66-67)

Vegetable oils are also damaging to the reproductive system and lungs. They are toxic to the liver and depress the immune system. They adversely affect growth in children. They inhibit the ability to learn.

They increase levels of uric acid in the blood. They contribute to obesity. They accelerate aging. They have been strongly linked to increasing rates of cancer and CVD. They inhibit the production of prostaglandins, leading to autoimmune diseases and menstrual difficulties. Decreased prostaglandin production also directly contributes to blood clot formation, the cause of myocardial infarction (Fallon and Enig, "Oiling," 9-10). In other words: ◆ *vegetable oils are bad news and you need to avoid them at all costs.* Check all labels of foods you buy, especially baked goods; do not purchase them if they contain vegetable oils.

The principal reason why vegetable oils are so harmful, besides how they are processed, is that, like white sugar and white flour, we humans did not evolve eating them. It is true that we've been eating corn for a long time, **but not isolated corn oil.** Our bodies are simply not equipped to handle them.

What should we use in their place? Traditional fats that have nourished people for a long time: olive oil, sesame oil, lard, butter, tallow, flax oil (do NOT heat this oil), coconut, and palm oil.

3. TRANS-FATTY ACIDS

Discussed in the last chapter, trans-fats are unnaturally shaped lipids that wreak havoc with our cells ability to function. These unnatural compounds are formed during the process of *hydrogenation*, the addition of hydrogen atoms to polyunsaturated vegetable oils. Margarine and vegetable shortening are the two largest sources of trans-fats in the Western diet. Like vegetable oils, ◆ *you need to avoid these two synthetic products like the plagues they cause.* Most people are unaware exactly how margarine is made. Here is a detailed and graphic description from Sally Fallon:

To produce them [margarine and vegetable shortening], manufacturers begin with the cheapest oils-soy, corn, or cottonseed-already rancid from the extraction process [described above]. These oils are then mixed with tiny metal particles, usually nickel oxide. Nickel oxide is very toxic when absorbed and is impossible to totally eliminate from margarine. The oil with its nickel catalyst is then subjected to hydrogen gas in a high pressure reactor. Next, soap-like emulsifiers and starch are squeezed into the mixture to give it a better consistency; the oil is yet again subjected to high temperature when it is steam-cleaned. This removes its horrible odor. Margarine's natural color, an unappetizing gray, is removed by bleach. Coal-tar dyes and strong flavors must then be added to make it resemble butter. Finally the mixture is compressed and packaged into blocks or tubs, ready to spread onto your toast. (*Nourishing Traditions,* 12)

Feel like eating some now? Doesn't butter sound like a great alternative? That's because it is.

Biochemically, trans-fats are just as bad as vegetable oils. Dr. Mary Enig, a lipid biochemist who has done more to call attention to the dangers of trans-fats than any other researcher, asserts that trans-fats raise Lp(a) levels, cause the loss of essential fatty acids from cells, interfere with many enzyme systems, including those that neutralize carcinogens, disrupt the immune system, and inhibit insulin binding, thus leading to blood sugar imbalances ("Fat Facts," 14; *Know Your Fats,* 86).

Other researchers have shown that trans-fats contribute to osteoporosis, decrease testosterone levels, cause abnormal sperm production, predispose women to give birth to low birth weight babies, and increase potential for cancer. With regards to CVD, Kummerow, Enig, and Mann all showed that ◆ *trans-fat consumption increases the incidence of heart disease* (See references in works cited).

Despite this, the food industry continues to manufacture margarine and shortening and establishment nutritionists recommend vegetable oil 'spreads" as better food choices than butter because, although spreads have trans-fats, they still contain no saturated fat (Tasker). Some food companies have even come out with trans-fat free spreads, usually made with canola oil. What they don't tell you is that canola oil is another new fangled fat, goes rancid easily, and causes vitamin E deficiencies in lab animals (Enig, "Fat Facts," 14).

The disturbing thing is that the food industry continues to assert that trans-fats are not harmful in small amounts, and that the typical Westerner consumes only a small amount from processed foods. Enig and her colleagues have shown otherwise and the industry has fought tooth and nail to silence them, as well as to discredit their findings.

One way it does this is by pointing out that butterfat has trans-fats in it. It is true, butter contains about 4% trans-veccenic acid. But once again, the difference here is one of natural versus synthetic. Ruminating animals convert most of this trans-fat into conjugated linoleic acid, a highly beneficial anti-carcinogen. The remaining small amounts are handled by humans without difficulty. There is little similarity, however, with a trans-fat artificially made from a vegetable oil. Such concoctions are new to our physiology and we cannot handle them.

The next step should be abundantly clear: discard all trans-fats from your life and never, never consume margarine.

4. PASTEURIZED AND HOMOGENIZED MILK

Though the evidence is not all in yet, there does seem to be a link between drinking commercially heated milk and heart disease. For example, a researcher named Annand discovered a correlation between heated milk protein and a tendency to form blood clots. He also noted that the rise in CVD in America began in the 1920s when laws requiring milk pasteurization went into effect (Fallon and Enig, "Diet and Heart Disease," 4).

Dr. William Campbell Douglass, MD, author of *The Milk Book,* a book that urges a return to raw milk and cream, also argues that homogenized milk causes atherosclerosis, citing research done by Oster. In the homogenization process, the fat particles in the cream are broken up by straining the fat through small pores under high pressures. The resulting fat particles are small enough to be absorbed by the intestines directly into the bloodstream, thus bypassing the lymphatic system. Oster contends that the fat molecules provide a vehicle for the transport of a harmful enzyme called XO, or xanthine oxidase which is not completely destroyed by pasteurization. Oster argues that the XO "sticks" to the fat molecules and then deposits itself in the arteries. Oster noted that such problems do not occur when milk is in its raw state and, therefore, unpasteurized and non-homogenized (Douglass, 103-107).

Dr. William Grant, Ph.D., has also been arguing that a large lactose intake (lactose is the sugar found in milk products) is a factor in atherosclerosis (*Nature's Impact*, 35-38). Grant notes, though, that when milk is fermented, the lactose is chemically transformed and little risk is involved. Fermented milk products include kefir, yogurt, piima, and cottage cheese. This might be the reason why most native peoples who consume milk products, ferment them, although there are exceptions to this rule. Fermented dairy, though, is much easier to digest than non-fermented as the process of lactofermentation "predigests" the nutrients in the milk. People who are lactose intolerant can usually handle fermented dairy.

Milk is a tragic example of how modern "food science" can destroy a supremely healthy food. When milk is raw, it is full of beneficial enzymes and easily assimilated nutrients. The minute that milk is pasteurized and homogenized, it is dead. The commercial milk sold in supermarkets is best avoided by everyone. It comes from cows which were bred to have abnormally large pituitary glands, thus forcing them to produce more milk. Additionally, at least in America, commercial dairy farmers are allowed to inject bovine growth hormone into their cows, artificially prompting them to produce more milk. The result is chronic mastitis; the commercial cow regularly secretes pus into her milk and must be given constant doses of antibiotics to stave off disease.

Given all of this unsettling information, its best to consume cheeses made from raw milk (readily available in health food markets—check the labels), whole milk organic yogurt (without added fruit—add your own), and cultured dairy products. If you can find a source of clean raw milk, or if you're able to own a Jersey cow, get your milk from there.

Bacterial contamination is usually the reason given to justify milk pasteurization, but with modern milking machines and stainless steel tanks, it is no longer necessary. In America, raw milk is legally sold in only two states—California and Georgia. Dairies that sell raw milk are held to high standards of cleanliness, much higher than dairies that pasteurize/ homogenize. There have been no reported outbreaks of disease from raw milk sold from these dairies, despite public health officials claims to the contrary. You should also know that one of the most common and serious food-borne diseases, salmonella, is unaffected by pasteurization. All milk-related salmonella outbreaks in America have been from pasteurized milk, not raw milk. For more on milk, visit www.realmilk.com.

4. OXIDIZED CHOLESTEROL

Found in products like powdered milk, powdered eggs, ultra high temperature (UHT) milk, and skim and low fat milk (which contain powdered milk), oxidized cholesterol is damaged cholesterol that might be dangerous to your arteries (Gittleman, 90, 190-191). The cholesterol used by Kritchevsky in his rabbit experiments was powdered, oxidized cholesterol. If you have such foodstuffs in your life, get rid of them quickly.

5. ALCOHOL AND CAFFEINE

Some researchers link excessive alcohol intake to heart disease. "A case-control study carried out to evaluate the relationship of alcohol to coronary heart disease in which the medical records of 568 married whites, who died from coronary heart disease, were matched with a corresponding control who were neighbors of the patients. Surprisingly, the results indicated that the daily use of a small amount of alcohol may result in a small decrease in coronary death, but they stressed that the seemingly beneficial effect was confined to light drinkers and definitely did not apply to heavy drinkers (Abrams, "Vegetarianism," 62). Although the link to heart disease is not 100%, alcohol does cause calcium loss from the bones. Alcohol, then, is a contributing factor in osteoporosis. Calcium is also required by the body to control blood pressure.

Excessive caffeine intake may also be a factor in heart disease. Caffeine stresses the adrenal glands and causes calcium loss. In high enough amounts, caffeine can lead to general exhaustion, including exhaustion of the heart muscle. Abrams cites studies which indicate excessive caffeine may lead to increased fatty substances in the blood, as well as irregular heart beat ("Beware of Coffee…," 22).

The best advice is moderation: restrict alcohol and caffeine intake.

NUTRITIONAL DEFICIENCIES

1. Vitamin C

Vitamin C deficiency makes for weaker arterial walls, subject to more inflammation and tearing (Fallon and Enig, "Diet and Heart Disease," 4). ◆*Adequate vitamin C intake, then, makes for stronger, healthier blood vessels and heart muscle.* How much is "adequate?" Dr. Linus Pauling, the king of vitamin C, recommends several grams a day which is well in excess of the recommended daily amount of 50-80 mgs (8). Since vitamin C is an antioxidant, it is reasonable to suppose that it would prevent oxidative damage to blood vessels. Pauling contends that an increased intake of vitamin C could reduce mortality from CVD for at risk people by 20 to 60% (199).

Vitamin C is the one vitamin not made by our bodies, so we must get our supply from our food. Raw milk, acerola powder and fresh fruits and vegetables are our best sources. Certain types of blubber also contain appreciable amounts. This is how the Eskimo get theirs, but its unlikely that any of us will be chowing down on blubber any time soon! For us, its better to eat a few servings of fruits and vegetables each day AND supplement with acerola powder to insure we get enough each day. Vitamin C is involved in so many biochemical processes that its too important to overlook. There is no danger from consuming an excess of vitamin C, so why not start supplementing today?

2. Mineral

According to Fallon and Enig, "Heart disease has been correlated with mineral deficiencies. Coronary heart disease rates are lower in regions where drinking water is naturally rich in trace minerals, particularly magnesium, which acts as a natural anti-coagulant and aids potassium absorption, thereby preventing heartbeat irregularities ("Diet and Heart Disease," 4).

Other minerals required by the cardiovascular system are iodine, needed for a healthy thyroid (poor thyroid function is a major factor in heart disease), calcium, chromium, selenium, and potassium. Calcium and potassium help to maintain proper blood pressure. Calcium and magnesium work together to maintain the health of the muscular system and the heart is, after all, a muscle. Selenium deficiencies have been linked to heart disorders (Lieberman and Bruning, 173). Chromium, through its ability to control and lower blood insulin levels, indirectly benefits the heart.

The best food sources for minerals are organic butter, raw nuts, sea foods, organ meats, dark green leafy vegetables, and cultured dairy products such as yogurt and cheese. Mineral supplements are readily available over the counter at health food stores. Always choose a complete mineral supplement, preferably one with added vitamin D and hydrochloric acid to assist with calcium absorption. Other supplement options include kelp and/or alfalfa tablets, and azomite mineral powder (see the Resources Section in the back for information).

One word of caution—those of you eating a diet high in whole grains, legumes, or nuts need to take steps to properly prepare these foods to avoid mineral malabsorption—calcium, iron, and zinc especially. Phytic acid is an organic acid found in the bran of all grains, as well as seeds, nuts, and legumes. Phytic acid binds to minerals in the digestive tract, thereby preventing their absorption in the intestines. To neutralize the phytates, simply soak your chosen grain, nut, legume, or seed in lightly salted water at room temperature for at least seven hours before cooking. The water initiates the chemical breakdown of the phytates and other antinutrients. Soaking will also render these foods more digestible—it is similar to sprouting. Soaking seed foods is a very common practice in traditional diets, as is fermentation.

3. Folate, B6, and B12

Researcher Kilmer McCulley has found a positive relationship between deficiencies in these three B vitamins and atherosclerosis, as well as buildup of arterial plaque. Because Westerners are consuming so much devitalized foods, these B vitamins, along with riboflavin, are often lacking in people's diets. B6 and B12 are primarily found in animal products—the very ones that the Lipid Hypothesis tells us to avoid! Folic acid is found in dark green leafy vegetables, but is very plentiful in liver, just like B6 and B12. Because of the unjustified cholesterol scare, people have shied away from liver, a supremely healthy food. If you like liver, then, make room for it a few times a month. B complex supplements are also an option, but I always recommend supplements as additions to good food, not replacements.

These three nutrients also lower levels of **homocysteine**, an amino acid that can trigger heart disease. McCulley has authored an entire book, *The Homocysteine Revolution* (Keats Publishing, Inc; 1997), explaining his theory as to how this amino acid contributes to heart disease and how these three B vitamins can correct the problem. McCulley points out that another B vitamin, **choline** (plentiful in eggs), helps convert homocysteine to methionine, an essential amino acid, and that choline deficiency contributes to increased homocysteine levels and atherosclerosis (Gazella, 3).

4. Antioxidants

"Oxidative stress" is the term given to an insidious condition whose effects are seen over time. It occurs when the body's available supply of antioxidants is insufficient to handle the amount of free radical stressors in the body. Free radicals are unstable molecules that attack and destroy cells, DNA, tissues, enzymes, and arterial walls. They have conclusively been shown to be causative/contributing factors in a growing list of diseases: cancer, lupus, rheumatoid arthritis, AIDS, Parkinson's, Alzheimer's, chronic pulmonary disease, diabetes mellitus, and atherosclerosis.

Where do free radicals come from? The body produces some as a part of everyday living. When a cell burns glucose for fuel, it oxidizes the sugar and free radicals are part of the by-products of that metabolism. The liver also uses free radicals to detoxify harmful substances from our bodies (drugs, chemicals, insecticides, food preservatives and colorings, etc). Surprisingly, our white blood cells use free radicals to attack and destroy invading organisms.

The other source is our environment and our food. By far, the largest source of free radicals is vegetable oils damaged by heat and transfatty acids. As noted earlier, heat, light, and oxygen damage and break down fats. Polyunsaturates are particularly susceptible to attack due to their more fragile chemical structure. Every time that you eat a bag of potato chips, some canned nuts, or some french fries from a local fast food place, you are eating millions of free radicals that, over time, can degenerate and destroy your body and its systems.

Other sources of free radicals are tobacco smoke, drugs (legal or illegal), unnatural chemicals, pollution, radiation (even from sunlight), and excessive exercise. Even psychological and emotional stress generates free radical formation by the body. During the stress response, the body produces certain hormones which the liver must detoxify. In that process, free radicals are created.

Although the body maintains a sophisticated system of anti-oxidants to neutralize free radicals, our hectic, malnourished, pollution-filled lives can overwhelm the body's defenses. It is, therefore, advisable to ingest as many antioxidants as possible, especially if one smokes or lives in a high-pollution area. The main antioxidants are glutathione peroxidase (GSH), superoxide dismutase (SOD), catalase, alpha lipoic acid, plant carotenes, vitamin C, vitamin E, selenium, zinc, vitamin A, ubiquinone (CoQ10), and various compounds found in assorted vegetables and herbs.

Whole foods are a great source of antioxidants. Try to include the following in your diet: dark green leafy vegetables (carotenes), seafood (zinc, vitamin A, selenium), fresh meats (glutathione, CoQ10, selenium, zinc), butter (selenium, vitamins A and E), orange and yellow fruits/vegetables (carotenes, vitamin C), organ meats like liver and heart (vitamin A, zinc, vitamin D, CoQ10, glutathione), green tea (polyphenols), and spices like curry and turmeric.

Supplements are your next best source. Since there is no one anti-oxidant that will neutralize all free radicals, its better to take a combination, or "cocktail," of antioxidants for a more complete effect. Look for a combination supplement, available at any health food store. One can also add herbs like milk thistle and ginkgo biloba into one's supplement regime. Low-heat, dried whey protein powder is an excellent and inexpensive supplement to safely raise one's glutathione levels—the key antioxidant of the liver.

5. Vitamins A & D

First put forward by Dr. Weston Price, deficiencies of these vital fat-soluble vitamins may be causes of heart disease. Dr. Price noticed that heart attack rates were higher in areas in the winter when available butter supplies had lower amounts of these vitamins. Conversely, heart attack rates dropped in the summer months when butter from grass-fed cows was more available ("Note From Yesteryear" 19-24).

Though Price's theories have never been tested in a clinical setting, vitamin A is required for numerous bodily functions, including protein and mineral utilization and the uptake of iodine by the thyroid gland. Since poor thyroid function is a cause of heart disease, a deficiency could be an indirect cause of heart disease. Since vitamin D is needed for calcium utilization, a deficiency may cause increased calcification of the arteries, leading to accelerated atherosclerosis (Sullivan 52-61).

More research is needed here to be sure. If the theory is true, however, this could be the most serious indictment of the low-fat diet which is automatically low in vitamins a and d due to its de-emphasis on animal fats.

The best advice here is to consume whole foods rich in these nutrients: salmon, fish roe, liver, butter, and cod liver oil. Cod liver oil used to be a standard supplement in western countries and it needs to be again. It is rich in vitamins A and D, as well as Omega-3 fatty acids which are usually lacking in "civilized" diets. (see last chapter for more on EFAs).

LIFE-STYLE FACTORS

1. Smoking

Most everyone knows that smoking is not good for the body so I won't go into too much detail here. As a former smoker (two packs a day for 18 years), I can only tell you that, if you do smoke, it is possible to quit. It took me nine tries, but I finally did it through acupuncture and visualization. My breathing difficulties, constant mucous, and chest pains provided incentives as well. Since the nicotine in tobacco constricts the blood vessels, the heart has to pump much harder to get blood to the body when you smoke. Also, since cigarette smoke contains carbon monoxide, oxygen intake goes down, which means the heart has to pump that much harder to get oxygen to the body. Smoking also destroys vitamin C, needed for healthy arteries, and greatly increases oxidative reactions in the body, leading to atherosclerosis and cancer.

Your best bet is to quit. If you can't (or won't), then at least cut down. When I was gearing up to quit, I began to cut down to ease my withdrawal. I made a rule which I've found helps smokers really cut down: don't smoke when you're inside of anything. This means you will refrain from smoking in your house or your car, a restaurant, a bar or club, someone else's house, etc. If you force yourself to go outside each time you want a smoke, often you'll put it off as its too much trouble. This helps you to reduce.

2. Obesity

When you weigh too much, the heart is under greater strain to pump blood through the body. Over time, the heart gets burned out, especially since most obese people don't exercise, which strengthens the heart. Some people have great difficulty losing weight, but it can be done. You don't have to look like Mel Gibson or Rachel Ward, but you can certainly lose something. Since diets don't work and food reeducation is in order to successfully lose weight and keep it off, I suggest enlisting the help of a professional trained in nutrition. As one of those professionals, I've found that if people can just make the effort to eliminate sugar and alcohol from their diets, they will quickly lose several excessive pounds. I've had patients give up sugar, but replace their sugary snacks with such high caloric, but non-sweet, foods like nuts and plain yogurt and lose 20-30 pounds in a few months. They are always flabbergasted!

If you need to lose a few pounds, see your health professional for a checkup to get the go ahead for exercise and then get to a nutritional counselor for help in designing a weight loss program. These two things should help you lose, and also spare your heart a lot of strain.

3. Stress

Last, but not least, stress is a major factor in promoting virtually every illness. "Oxidative stress" is the new buzzword in the health community. It refers to the body's increasing depletion of antioxidant nutrients, thus allowing free radical degeneration to slowly but surely undermine the body's various systems, including the heart (see section on "Antioxidants" above).

At the risk of sounding like a New Age guru, it really does pay to go for a walk on the beach to unwind, to shut off the phone for a few hours and watch a good film or read, to rent some comedy videos and have a good laugh, to take short weekend getaways to relax, and to spend quality time with those you love. All these things release stress. If you are so inclined, you can take up meditation, proven time and again to lower blood pressure and relieve stress.

Using myself as an example, before I became a naturopath, I was working for a large hotel chain as a credit manager. Although I was well paid and the job was relatively easy, I had to work with two of the most despicable people I'd ever met in my life. It was truly "hate on sight" for me and them. For almost two years, I dreaded going in to work. My coworkers and I rarely spoke to each other, preferring to send emails even though we sat within three feet of each other! They would complain and bicker about me to management. I would defend myself and counter-complain. They would make fun of my mannerisms, but without naming me so I could never actually accuse them of anything.

What kept me going in? The money. I was finished with my training, but kept working there for the money. After all, to go into practice meant giving up that nice paycheck, and being in business for oneself is not easy, especially in the beginning. Deep down, however, it was what I always wanted. But I kept rationalizing my staying there. It was not a good decision.

During those two years, my relationship kept getting worse and worse. I was always on edge when I was at home. When I played tennis, I was very keyed up. I also got very sick with candidiasis and insomnia—all because I didn't have the guts to say, "I quit."

When I finally looked at my life and where it had gone, I thought, "Well this isn't life. I'm not enjoying it. What am I so afraid of?" I quit on my birthday. The day I walked out of there for the last time, I had no idea where my next paycheck was coming from, but I was smiling, and things did work out for me.

Only you can determine what stresses you the most. If its your job, then find another one or find a way to deal with what you have. If its a relationship, try to work on it with your partner and if they refuse, leave. If you have old guilts festering away at you, resolve them. If you've got skeletons in your closet, hidden fears, poor self-image, then face them once and for all. The decision to improve your life starts with just that—a decision. For many of us, that is the hardest step. It is a step, however, that must be taken for our well being.

MISCELLANEOUS CAUSES

Heart disease can arise from a number of lesser known and less frequent causes such as syphilis and other infectious diseases, whether of bacterial, vial, or fungal origin. Certain toxins, like carbon monoxide and drugs, can also damage the heart. Autoimmune diseases, including rheumatoid arthritis and lupus, also factor in. Let us also not overlook congenital birth or genetic defects, as well. These causes, compared to our current dietary ones, are less frequent to be sure, but must still be taken into consideration. Since many of us live in cities, and since cities have smog which can cause increased free radical production and oxidation in the body, we could all benefit from either (1) taking a strong multivitamin/mineral rich in antioxidants, or (2) moving away from the smog (or both!).

Fallon and Enig rightly point out, however, that, "Heart disease due to syphilis and infectious disease has been around for a long time and probably accounts for a good portion of CHD deaths before 1920" ("Diet and Heart Disease," 4).

KEY POINTS TO REMEMBER

◆ *Wherever refined sugar goes, dental decay and disease follow.*

◆ *Heat, light, and oxygen damage oils and denature them, eventually turning them rancid.*

◆ *All deep fried foods fried in vegetable oil or shortening should be strictly avoided; this includes commercially roasted nuts.*

◆ *Vegetable oils are bad news and you need to avoid them at all costs.*

◆ *You need to avoid these two synthetic products, margarine and shortening, like the plagues they cause.*

◆ *Trans-fat consumption increases the incidence of heart disease.*

◆ *Adequate vitamin C intake makes for stronger, healthier blood vessels and heart muscle.*

CHAPTER FIVE

Hypothyrodism: A Little Known—But Deadly—Cause

The thyroid gland is a small part of the endocrine system that straddles the front part of the neck. Most anatomy and physiology texts state that this little gland helps to regulate one's overall energy levels, blood sugar, body temperature, and, through its action on the parathyroid glands, blood calcium levels. But there is much more.

There are two medical conditions associated with the thyroid: **hyperthyroidism** and **hypothyroidism**. In hyperthyroidism, one's metabolism is speeded up and assorted physical symptoms occur: bulging eyes, weight loss, increased nervousness, diarrhea, increased sweating, feeling hot, hair loss, less frequent menstruation, hand tremors, and rapid heartbeat. It is less common than its more dangerous twin, hypothyroidism.

In this condition, the thyroid under secretes its two hormones with disastrous effects. The symptoms of hypothyroidism are more vague and therefore more difficult to diagnose—physical weakness, dry skin, lethargy, slow speech, swelling of face or eyelids, coldness and cold skin, diminished sweating, thickened tongue, coarse hair, pale skin, constipation, weight gain, hair loss, difficult breathing, swollen feet, hoarseness, poor appetite, excessive or painful menstruation, nervousness, depression, emotional instability, heart palpitations, high blood pressure, poor memory, sexual dysfunction, and headaches. Another unfortunate effect of too little thyroid hormone is the loss of the body's ability to convert carotenes into vitamin A in the small intestines.

69

With such a varied list, ◆ *it is easy for your typical medical practitioner to misdiagnose the problem.* Its important to point out here that not everyone with hypothyroidism will manifest ALL of these symptoms. Some may show a few, while others may show many; it all depends on the individual. A typical misdiagnosis is hypoglycemia, or low blood sugar. If you suspect hypothyroidism, then, your health provider should rule this condition out first to be sure you really have a thyroid problem.

The problem, however, in diagnosing hypothyroidism is that most medical tests won't show anything abnormal, yet the problem is still there. naturopaths will typically rely on a number of techniques to ascertain if the thyroid is stressed or not, not just a blood hormone level result. One of the most used analytical methods is iris analysis, or iridology. The naturopath will typically check the area at about 2:30 in the right iris, and 9:30 in the left for any markings or discolorations. If something shows there, there is a good chance that something is amiss.

Another technique used is reflex analysis. In reflexology, the nerve endings of all of the body's organs and areas are present, by reflex action, in the feet. The thyroid is located at the base of the big toe on the sole side. An additional area is around the ball of the foot. If these areas are tender or sensitive to pressure, it is, again, an indication that something is amiss. Other techniques of diagnosis could be Touch for Health and Applied Kinesiology. Personally, I always recommend reflexology to my patients as anyone can do it, you just need to know where to press.

If you have some of the symptoms I've listed above, you should definitely explore the possibility that you might have hypothyroidism, take appropriate action, and enlist the help of a qualified naturopath (see the Resources Section to locate a suitably trained Doctor of Naturopathy) for resolution; an underactive thyroid can be hard on your heart and arteries.

THE THYROID AND CVD

Over a hundred years ago in London, a medical task force was organized to investigate a seemingly new disease wherein the affected people would have a grossly enlarged, fibrous thyroid gland, mucin-logged tissues, a tight-skinned, mask-like face and severe atherosclerosis. A 300 page report followed showing that the condition was caused by an under functioning thyroid gland.

In 1890, in Vienna, Austria, pathologists discovered that thyroid insufficiency helped to bring on heart attacks. At the time, no one paid much attention to these results as heart disease was a rare occurrence. Nevertheless, science continued to investigate the role of the thyroid in relation to the heart. They discovered that if the thyroid gland was re-moved from test animals, they subsequently developed mucin-logged tis-sues and severe atherosclerosis (Langer and Scheer, 108). When doctors performed the thyroidectomy on patients, due to life-threatening goiter, they too developed atherosclerosis and died soon after the operation.

Years later, two Viennese doctors began giving thyroid extract to their patients who had received thyroidectomies, thinking that perhaps it would avert their deaths. They were right. British physicians learned that Chinese doctors for thousands of years had given "thyroid soup" to weakened patients to rejuvenate them. The British doctors began serving raw animal thyroid sandwiches to their patients to good effect. Unfortunately, most patients found the food unpalatable and eventually the doctors found a way to dry out the fresh animal thyroid, creating a desiccated thyroid product. The product worked like a charm for virtually all patients who took it. Their thyroid diffi-culties disappeared and with them, all of the secondary symptoms, including the atherosclerosis and heart troubles (Langer and Scheer, 109-110). The physician who developed the preparation, Dr. G.R. Murray, popularized the use of desiccated thyroid for thyroid-related heart problems.

Unfortunately, because of the heavy promotion of the Lipid Hy-pothesis as the principal cause of CVD, Dr. Murray's work, as well as the work of other physicians who have discovered the wonders of thyroid treatment, remains mostly forgotten. One wonders how many people died of atherosclerosis or heart attacks on a useless low-fat/cholesterol diet, when all they might have needed was some desiccated thyroid!

Apparently, ◆ *when there is no thyroid hormone, or not enough of it, triglycerides (blood fats) begin accumulating in the blood in very high amounts,* eventually causing occlusions and heart attacks. Blood cholesterol levels also rise to skyrocketing proportions.

No one has done more to re-popularize the thyroid treatment ap-proach than Dr. Broda Barnes. Barnes has had nothing but success us-ing desiccated thyroid for his diabetic patients who develop circulatory problems or diabetic retinopathy, caused by a breakdown of the blood vessels in the eyes. Of course, Barnes also uses the preparation for hypothyroidal patients, also to good effect.

Thyroid extracts are available either in health food stores or through Natural Therapists. Due to some evidence that too much thyroid supple-mentation can lead to dangerous complications, its best to use it under the supervision of a health professional. Another option, one that I use with my patients who are hypothyroidal, is a homeopathic preparation called *Thyroidinum*, homeopathic thyroid. I've found the 6C potency to work best. If you are unable to acquire desiccated thyroid, or are afraid to use it, you can try the homeopathic approach; it may work for you.

THINGS THAT DEPRESS THYROID FUNCTION

Iodine deficiency is one that most people know, yet, iodized salt does not prevent thyroid problems. Iodine will only prevent one type of disorder: goiter. Langer and Scheer note several causes of thyroid depression. Among them are fluoridated tap water, certain drugs such as barbiturates, sulfa, anti-diabetic medications, aspirin, some cough medicines, lithium, and nicotine from tobacco products (37-38).

Certain foods, known as *goitrogens*, can inhibit thyroid function by blocking the uptake of iodine, required to synthesize thyroid hormones. Foods such as cabbage, kale, turnips, peaches, pears, cauliflower, mustard greens, and millet, if consumed to excess, can depress thyroid function. Cooking, or lactofermentation, usually inactivates the goitrogens, but in cases of severe hypothyroidism, its probably best to avoid them altogether until you're out of the woods.

One food that powerfully inhibits thyroid function is soy. ◆ *Several studies have demonstrated that soybeans and soy foods depress thyroid function* (summarized in Fitzpatrick, 3-6). I am not a fan of soy products, despite the warm reviews they receive from both the medical and holistic communities. There is a mountain of research, carefully kept from the public, that suggests that soy may not be all that it is cracked up to be. For those of you interested in reading more about this, you can log onto the following web site, **www.soyonlineservice.co.nz** and/or **www.westonaprice.org** for information on soy's darker side. Fermented soy products (miso, tempeh, and natto), are better choices than unfermented ones (soy milk, "cheese," textured vegetable protein, and tofu) as the fermentation process effectively breaks down soy's considerable enzyme inhibitors; cooking does not do the job (Fallon and Enig, "Soy Products..."). Most people are unaware that Asians did not begin consuming soybeans, even though they grew them, until they learned how to ferment them. In any event, because of its proven deleterious effect on the thyroid gland, soy consumption should not be excessive and, if one has hypothyroidism, it must be avoided completely.

THINGS THAT KEEP THE THYROID HAPPY

◆ *First and foremost is vitamin A.* Without vitamin A, all of the endocrine glands will suffer. Without vitamin A, the body cannot properly utilize proteins, also required for a healthy thyroid. I need to emphasize here that beta-carotene, available in yellow and orange vegetables and fruits, is NOT the same thing as vitamin A; this is one of the biggest nutritional myths going today. Beta carotene is a precursor to vitamin A and the body carries out the conversion in the upper portion of the small intestines with the help of thyroid hormone, bile, and fat. If one has a thyroid or gall bladder problem, the conversion cannot take place. If one is diabetic or alcoholic, the conversion cannot take place. If one is an infant, the conversion cannot take place. Assuming you're not in one of these groups, you now have to realize that the body's conversion from carotene to vitamin A is inefficient: it takes six units of betacarotene to make one unit of vitamin A. Relying on plant sources, then, for your vitamin A requirement is not a wise idea.

Isobel Jennings, in her classic *Vitamins and Endocrine Metabolism*, cites studies showing that vitamin A deficiency severely limits the body's ability to manufacture TSH (thyroid stimulating hormone), and interferes with the thyroid's ability to utilize iodine.

The people most likely to suffer from a vitamin A-related thyroid problem are those who practice strict vegetarianism, vegans. Langer and Scheer cite numerous case histories of vegans suffering from hypothyroidism due to inadequate vitamin A and protein (27-31). In my own files, I have a few as well. This is one of the reasons why butter is such an important addition to the diet. It contains easily absorbed vitamin A (and all the other fat-soluble vitamins), as well as iodine. Placed on vegetables, it provides the fatty material needed by the intestines to convert carotenes into vitamin A. Cod liver oil is also an excellent supplemental source of vitamin A.

The B complex are also needed as well, especially riboflavin (B2), niacin (B3), and pyrodoxine (B6). Barnes noted the increased effectiveness of desiccated thyroid when he administered it with Brewer's yeast tablets, rich in the B vitamins (Langer and Scheer, 23).

◆ *Without a proper functioning thyroid, we cannot efficiently absorb vitamin B12* (Langer and Scheer, 32). This nutrient is available only from animal products. Plant foods do not contain it. It is true that there are vitamin B12 analogs in such foods as tempeh (a soy product) and spirulina (an algae), but it is in a form not usable by the body. Vegans, therefore, are doubly at risk, not only for thyroid insufficiency, but also for vitamin B12 deficiency, a very serious and life-threatening condition. Remember that B12 is needed to control homocysteine levels (see last chapter).

Langer and Scheer also point out that vitamins C and E are depleted rapidly when hyperthyroidism is present (34). Sufficient amounts of these vitamins must be ingested daily to avoid problems.

Two other nutrients required by the thyroid are tyrosine, an amino acid that is part of thyroid hormone, and essential fatty acids. ◆ *Tyrosine deficiency, in particular, has been noted in hypothyroidism.* Luckily, it is easily available, either from a Natural Therapist or from a health food market. I have had great success using tyrosine with my patients with chronic fatigue syndrome and fibromyalgia, who frequently have thyroid and adrenal insufficiencies. Tyrosine is also a part of several adrenal hormones and promotes mental alertness. A side benefit is that it suppresses appetite. So if you're looking to lose weight...

Foods that stimulate thyroid function are molasses, eggs, parsley, apricots, dates, and prunes. Raw milk cheeses are also a good addition.

THE BARNES SELF-THYROID TEST

Dr. Barnes developed a fast and easy way to determine if your thyroid is under functioning. If you suspect hypothyroidism, do the following test for five consecutive days. If you are a woman, avoid doing this test when you're menstruating:

Keep a thermometer by your bed. When you wake up in the morning, place the thermometer under your arm by your armpit and leave it there for 15 minutes. Do not move or speak for the 15 minutes as it may upset the reading. Now, read your temperature. If it is LESS than 97.6° F, it is a good indication that something is amiss and you should see your health care professional.

Just as modern medicine under recognizes hypothyroidism, it also leads people to think that it can safely monitor and handle heart problems by using certain tests and procedures, as well as drugs.

KEY POINTS TO REMEMBER

◆ *It is easy for your typical medical practitioner to misdiagnose the problem.*

◆ *When there is no thyroid hormone, or not enough of it, triglycerides (blood fats) begin accumulating in the blood in very high amounts.*

◆ *Several studies have demonstrated that soybeans and soy foods depress thyroid function.*

◆ *First and foremost is vitamin A for maintaining a healthy thyroid.*

◆ *Without a proper functioning thyroid, we cannot efficiently absorb vitamin B12.*

◆ *Tyrosine deficiency, in particular, has been noted in hypothyroidism.*

CHAPTER SIX

EKG's, Bypass, Angioplasty, & Other Non-Solutions

The medical world's standard solutions for heart disease consist of dietary modification (which we've already seen to be faulty), drugs, and a battery of surgical and testing procedures of little value. Its important to realize that a clean bill of health from an MD does not necessarily mean that one's heart is healthy.

EKG's

Also known as an "electrocardiogram," this test claims to be able to detect heart disease, but "most doctors have files on patients documenting completely normal EKG's hours before a fatal heart attack. The EKG will only detect heart disease in 10 to 20 percent of future victims. The stress EKG (e.g., using a treadmill) will detect 10 to 15 percent more. It is only when heart disease is advanced and, often too late, that the EKG shows the abnormality. In other words, the EKG may be normal but the patient is dead" (Rona, 6).

What this obviously boils down to is that ◆ *a normal EKG does not mean you're OK.* You also need to know that up to 25% of routine EKG screenings are falsely positive (Rona, 6). If you receive an EKG, then, be wary of the results. Far better to gauge your heart's health using other methods.

ANGIOGRAMS

An angiogram attempts to assess whether a coronary artery is blocked. If there is a positive result, a bypass operation is recommended.

But, as Dr. Zoltan Rona, MD, points out, "Since an angiogram cannot image the small arteries that make up the heart's microcirculation, this procedure results in over-diagnosis and unnecessary surgery" (6). In other words, the procedure is virtually worthless.

BYPASS OPERATIONS

Bypass surgery consists of rerouting blood flow around blockages by grafting in a piece of vein taken from elsewhere in the body (Rowland, 1). Bypass surgery can only be performed on parts that are accessible to the surgeon's scalpel. The back of the heart, for example, is unavailable for bypass for this reason.

The medical world pushes bypass operations and they are a very big business. Unfortunately, ◆ *the effectiveness of the procedure has NEVER been validated by any type of clinical study.* If you compare those who have had the operation to those who have not, the procedure "does nothing to extend life. Those who have bypass surgery, on the average, do not live longer than those in similar condition who do not" (Rowland, 1). The *New England Journal of Medicine* (11/08/88) reported the dismal results of a study of 767 European men at several European hospitals. Of the 767, 109 who had the procedure died within twelve years, as opposed to 92 in the group that did not have it. Moreover, 34 men had to have the operation performed again, and five of these died.

Risks from bypass operations are many. They include migrating blood clots leading to possible strokes, blurred vision, and loss of consciousness (Rowland, 2). A small percentage of patients die on the operating table (Ibid.).

With such a lousy track record, it is odd that bypass continues to be touted as the ideal solution to atherosclerosis. Far better alternatives (and less expensive ones, too) would be chelation therapy using an intravenous preparation of EDTA, a synthetic amino acid that gradually dissolves arterial plaque and removes it from the body. Another option, even less expensive, is the use of an Arterial Cleansing Formula composed of nutrients in exact proportions and ratios. Though slower acting than chelation, the formula, in clinical practice, has worked wonders for many people. If you're interested in this formula, please contact me through *WellBeing*, or my email (see Resources).

ANGIOPLASTY

Angioplasty is a less invasive surgical procedure than bypass. Basically, a balloon catheter is inserted into the blocked blood vessel, inflated, and then rubbed back and forth to expand the artery and mash the plaque against the arterial wall. A little thinking will show any rational person that the procedure does nothing to prevent additional plaque from forming on top of the compressed plaque, leading to an occluded artery.

As with bypass operations, studies indicate that the artery operated on gets blocked again, usually within six months after the procedure (Rowland, 3). As with heart bypass operations, this procedure does not get to the CAUSE of the blockages; therefore, the procedures are palliative at best and dangerous at worst. The procedure, however, does seem to lessen angina pains in some patients, making it of some value. The ultimate problem, though, is not addressed by the operation.

CHOLESTEROL TESTING

We saw in chapter four that lowering cholesterol levels has no positive impact on heart disease as cholesterol has never been proven to cause heart disease or heart attacks. If a high cholesterol reading is obtained, invariably, the patient will be told to stop eating saturated fats, animal products (again, worthless advice as we have seen) and take cholesterol-lowering drugs, drugs that have very unpleasant side effects (see below). The public is often not told that ◆ *low cholesterol levels are associated with increased cancer risk and immune disorders* (Rona, 5). We also saw in chapter four that low cholesterol levels correlate strongly with depression and violent behavior. This is also not told to the public.

Numerous things can elevate blood cholesterol levels: poor thyroid function, smoking, stress, sedentary behavior, refined sugars, and excessive alcohol intake are the main ones. Usually, these things are not addressed by medical practitioners, and they should be.

◆ *The principal reason why cholesterol levels are elevated is that there is excessive free radical activity in the body.* Free radicals damage cells and tissues, including those of the arteries. The body, in response to the greater damage to the blood vessels, secretes more cholesterol in an attempt to quell and repair the damage. Remember that cholesterol is an antioxidant.

CHOLESTEROL LOWERING DRUGS

Drugs that lower cholesterol levels are known to have a host of unpleasant side effects. For example, in the drug-treated groups in most heart disease studies, there were significantly higher rates of death by suicide and violence. Furthermore, apes given the same drugs acted more violently than apes who did not take them and that low cholesterol levels were often observed in criminals and people with a history of violent behavior and poor self-control (Muldoon, Manuck, and Matthews 309-314). Other researchers from Sweden and America have concluded that drug-induced low cholesterol levels cause violent behavior (Lindberg, et. al., 277-279; Golomb 478-487). Ravnskov also notes that deaths from cerebral hemorrhage are significantly higher in those with low cholesterol levels, including the Japanese who have the highest rates of this disorder in the world—something never mentioned by lipid hypothesis proponents (232-233).

Ravnskov also points out that the newer "Statin" drugs, hailed as miracle substances that prevent heart disease, lower choleterol levels and reverse athersclerosis, have caused cancer in lab animals and that women on the drugs in past trials have statistically significant higher breast cancer rates than those who did not take them (208-210). Statin drugs also appear to inhibit the body's production of Coenzyme Q10, a vital antioxidant needed by the heart for proper functioning.

The claims for Statin drugs are questionable also in light of Ravnskov's analysis of the data (198-213). These drugs are always recommended by doctors to those with "elevated" cholesterol levels. Though they may have some value for short-term use, do you really want to be taking something that could cause you cancer in the future, or that inhibits bodily production of a substance needed for energy production and a healthy heart?

Similar things could be said of hormone replacement therapy (HRT), advocated by most doctors to prevent heart disease in post-memopausal women. In an editorial published in the August/September 2000 issue of The Townsend Letter for Doctors, Alan Gaby, MD, critically analyzed the data supposedly proving HRT to prevent heart disease and found it wanting: "The evidence that HRT prevents heart disease has never been strong" (108). The increased cancer risks of HRT, however, are quite well known.

KEY POINTS TO REMEMBER

◆ *A normal EKG does not mean you're OK.*

◆ *The effectiveness of bypass has NEVER been validated by any type of clinical study.*

◆ *Low cholesterol levels are associated with increased cancer risk and immune disorders.*

◆ *The principal reason why cholesterol levels are elevated is that there is excessive free radical activity in the body.*

CHAPTER SEVEN

A Grab Bag of Good Things for Your Heart

If you are faced with a heart problem, it is best to be working with a qualified health professional rather than self-medicating yourself with the information in this chapter. Do not discontinue any medications without the approval of your health care provider. ◆*A naturopathic doctor or nutritional consultant can be a very useful complement to conventional allopathic therapy* and, in some cases, can be an adequate replacement for standard therapy. Remember that your health choices are just that--yours. You need to take the reins of your own recovery and your own health; our well being is our own responsibility, not someone else's.

HERBS

◆*Herbalists through the ages have long known of several plants that act favorably on the heart muscle and circulatory system.* Cayenne, peppermint, hawthorne berry, motherwort, lily of the valley, and gotu kola are the foundations, either singly or in combination, of any sound cardiac program. Of course, nutritional therapy is also of prime importance here with an emphasis on the vitamins C, E, and P (bioflavonoids), and the minerals calcium and magnesium. Let us now go through our herbs and see what they have to offer.

CAYENNE PEPPER: Famous American herbalist and naturopath, Dr. John Christopher, advocated this herb for a variety of ailments, but specifically for heart and circulatory troubles. Cayenne is a cardiac stimulant and a catalyst for other herbs, prompting them to act more powerfully. Christopher advocated giving 1 teaspoon of cayenne powder in a cup of warm water to quell a heart attack or stroke. Cayenne also helps with poor circulation and varicose veins as the herb acts to "elasticize" and strengthen blood vessels. Cayenne is of value in normalizing blood pressure, whether high or low. Lastly, cayenne is rich in several nutrients making it an ideal addition to one's daily diet. Peppers, however, are a known food allergen. Be sure you're not allergic to it before you take it.

PEPPERMINT: The famous *Handbook of Alternatives to Chemical Medicine* by Lawton and Teague recommends one cup of strong peppermint tea a day as a heart attack preventive. Like cayenne, peppermint is a stimulant herb, but with a more generalized action on the entire body. Peppermint's main chemical constituent is menthol which helps the blood carry oxygen more efficiently. It is this quality that makes peppermint valuable for treating headaches and migraines. Peppermint strengthens the nerves and myocardium and is good for heart palpitations. The most heavily used herb in the world, peppermint needs to be avoided if one is taking homeopathic remedies as the menthol in the herb can inactivate homeopathic medicines.

HAWTHORN BERRY: This is the most famous cardiac tonic, being the main herb prescribed by doctors before nitroglycerine. Hawthorn is the best remedy for heart and circulatory problems. Used for high and low blood pressure, angina pectoris, and arteriosclerosis, it is indicated for all functional heart disorders such as rapid and feeble heart action, valvular insufficiency, hypertrophy, myocarditis, pericarditis, cardiac dropsy, and extreme dyspnea on least exertion. Hawthorn's action is primarily to make the heart muscle contract more slowly, but also more forcefully. Over time, the heart muscle is strengthened. Hawthorn is also indicated for chilliness in the extremities, erratic pulse, and nervous prostration in heart failure. Unlike many herbs with strong medicinal properties, hawthorn is perfectly safe to use and may be taken for several months without any danger of overdosing.

MOTHERWORT: As its name implies, motherwort is primarily a women's herb being used to regulate the uterus in erratic periods, relax menstrual cramping, promote blood flow when the menses are delayed, and assist with the bodily changes of menopause. Motherwort is also a great pain reliever and antispasmodic. The herb is, along with hawthorn, the best cardiac tonic in the herbal world. Motherwort's actions are virtually identical to hawthorn's. Despite the bitter taste, motherwort is, like hawthorn, perfectly safe to take in large amounts for long periods of time.

GARLIC: Studied more than any other herb, garlic has been shown to prevent CVD, as well as to treat it. Garlic prevents platelet aggregation and, therefore, prevents blood clots and plaque accumulation on the arterial walls. In countries that consume a lot of garlic, such as Italy and Spain, atherosclerosis occurs less in the population (but other factors are involved as well). Garlic has long been used in herbal medicine for high blood pressure.

Since garlic has other health promoting properties, from cancer prevention to immune enhancement, it is a good herb to add to one's daily diet, either in food or as a supplement. Deodorized forms are available as supplements, reducing the notorious garlic smell that plagues users.

GOTU KOLA: Although this herb has no particular action on the heart, gotu kola is a well known peripheral vasodilator, helping with poor circulation to the extremities. Gotu kola also has a well-deserved reputation as a cerebral stimulant and assists with correcting brain fog, poor memory, and failing mental acuity.

One could make an excellent cardiac infusion by combining 2 oz (60 gms) of either hawthorn or motherwort, with 1 oz of either asparagus root or seed (a little known cardiac tonic, excellent for cardiac dropsy), and peppermint. Steep the herbs in 1 liter of very hot water, covered, for 20 minutes. Sweeten to taste if desired, cool, refrigerate, and take 2 ounces 3-4 times a day. For proper doses and herbs appropriate to your condition, its best to seek the advice of a qualified naturopath or herbal practitioner.

PADMA 28: Going by the name "Adaptrin" in the USA, Padma 28 is an ancient ayurvedic formula combining over 20 herbs and natural camphor with a number of uses. Since it was banned in the USA for many years by the U.S. Food and Drug Administration, there are few Americna studies verifying its effectiveness for health and circulatory problems. In Europe, however, where it has been freely sold andused for a very long time, several studies exist. for example, Polish researcher Brzosko showed that this compound is able to not only reduce serum level of Hepatitis B antigens, but also to increase the serum level of Hepatitis B antibodies (13-14). Since Padma 28 is rich in antioxidant nutrients, it helps curtail free radical activity, oxidative stress, and the inflammation these conditions cause. Dr. Alfred Hassig and his research colleagues specifically recommended Padma 28 as a safe and effective treatment for AIDS (along with other measures), poor circulation and CVD (July 1995). The Padma 28 formula is available in the United States from two companies: Pacific Biologic (Clayton, CA) and Padma Health Products (River Vale, NJ).

NUTRIENTS

In addition to the vitamins and minerals we discussed in chapter five, there are several nutrients that can help an ailing heart and circulatory system.

ANTIOXIDANTS: See the section on antioxidants in chapter five.

NIACIN: One of the B vitamins, niacin, or nicotinic acid, has a well-deserved reputation as a circulatory tonic. ◆ *Niacin is a vasodilator and increases peripheral circulation.* After taking it, you'll often feel flushed and itchy and your face will often turn bright red. This reaction, which lessens as you get used to the nutrient, occurs because niacin prompts the release of histamine from your mast cells, and also because it is dilating your capillaries. You'll often feel your blood pumping throughout your body a few minutes after taking niacin. It is this circulatory effect that makes niacin especially good for treating acne and arthritic pains. Ortho-molecular doctors use niacin to treat schizophrenia, depression, and cancer (Hoffer and Walker; Pauling; Lieberman and Bruning).

Since niacin plays a major role in fat metabolism, niacin is a safe treatment for lowering triglyceride levels in the bloodstream. You have to be sure that you're using real niacin (nicotinic acid), and not niacinamide, for this effect. Niacinamide, in very high amounts, has caused liver damage in some people and it does not possess the dilating qualities of true niacin. Studies have shown niacin to be more effective at lowering serum triglyceride levels than comparable prescription drugs (Lieberman and Bruning). Niacin is also cheap and, except for the flushing reaction, has no side effects.

Niacin is found in a wide variety of foods, mostly animal products—pork, eggs, milk, fish, and cheese, but is also found in whole wheat, potatoes, and carrots. Supplements are easily available over the counter.

A good starting dose for high TG levels would be 250-500 mg/day (Lieberman and Bruning), but a more accurate amount could be given by a naturopath or nutritionist (see Resources Section to locate a suitably trained practioner). Circulatory problems could best be approached by 100 mg/ three times a day. Time-release forms of niacin are not recommended. A newer form of niacin, called inositol hexaniacinate (IHN) is a flush-free form of niacin that may be used at high amounts with no adverse effects. Those of you with ulcers need to be careful with niacin supplementation as the nutrient prompts HCl release from the stomach.

VITAMIN E: The Shute brothers from Canada popularized the use of vitamin E for heart and circulatory problems in the 1960s and were ridiculed by the medical profession for it. Today, their work is increasingly verified. Vitamin E is one of the key antioxidants the body uses in preventing oxidation of lipids and the fat-soluble vitamins and it is important in the prevention of cancer and cardiovascular disease. It also improves circulation, as it is a natural blood thinner, and promotes normal blood clotting. Other uses for this vitamin include treatment of PMS and fibrocystic breasts, cataracts, and leg cramps. Vitamin E is also pivotal along with several other nutrients) for a healthy reproductive system and deficiencies have been linked to infertility.

Lieberman and Bruning report that practitioners have had considerable clinical success using vitamin E for angina, arteriosclerosis, poor circulation, and thrombophlebitis (79). In my experience, I have found this to be true.

Foods rich in vitamin E include fresh wheat germ, raw nuts, and whole grains. Vitamin E is present also in animal and vegetable fats, but in lesser amounts. Supplements are the preferred option if you want to add more into your diet. Always look for the "d-" form and not the "dl-" one. The "dl" is the synthetic one and is not as usable by the body. The Shute brothers used cold-pressed wheat germ oil in their studies, not isolated vitamin E supplements—something to consider when supplementing with this substance.

If you're currently taking anticoagulant medications, you should ask your doctor before supplementing with amount over 400 IUs per day. Also, if you have high blood pressure, you should begin supplementing with a lower dose (200 IU per day) and gradually work your way up to higher doses (800-1000 IU per day) as vitamin E can cause a temporary elevation of blood pressure. For CVD and poor circulation, though, a dose of 800-1200 IUs, divided throughout the day should be sufficient.

COENZYME Q10

Also called *ubiquinone*, this substance is similar in action to vitamin E and is found in mackerel, salmon, sardines, beef, liver, heart, peanuts, and spinach. The body also produces it, but production declines with age.

CoQ10 is intimately involved in energy production in our cellular mitochondria and is a standard supplement for people with chronic fatigue syndrome, fibromyalgia, and immune disorders. It is also used for treating allergies, asthma, muscular dystrophy, periodontal disease, and cancer. Ubiquinone is also a potent antioxidant and depressed levels are commonly seen in those suffering from oxidative stress and/or diseases associated with this condition (e.g., Parkinson's disease, AIDS, cancer, and CVD). Oxidative stress occurs when the body's pool of antioxidants are insufficient to handle its production of and exposure to free radicals.

Cardiovascular disease, however, is the main ailment benefited by CoQ10. The Japanese use the nutrient as a standard treatment for congestive heart failure and several large scale studies have shown CoQ10 to be extremely beneficial. Trials have also shown that CoQ10 is also of value in treating mitral valve prolapse, angina, and arrhythmias (Liberman and Bruning 187-191). One needs to realize, though, that *CoQ10 is not only appropriate for existing cardiovascular disorders, but also as a heart disease preventive as well.*

CoQ10 supplements are expensive so, for those of you with no heart disease, but looking to add more into your diet, foods are your best sources. For those with CVD, however, 50-200 mg per day appears to be a safe and effective dose. No side effects from larger doses have been reported, though.

ESSENTIAL FATTY ACIDS

EPA (eicosapentaenoic acid) and GLA (gamma linoleic acid) are two omega 3 and 6 fatty acids that are most used to treat and prevent heart disease. Many studies have shown that EPA protects against heart disease as it is a natural blood thinner and, therefore, prevents plaque and clot formation; GLA has been shown to have these properties as well. Both EPA and GLA help to normalize blood pressure and EPA, like niacin, is effective at lowering blood triglyceride levels, a possible factor in CVD (Lieberman and Bruning 192-197).

Because of the over consumption of vegetable oils in the Western world, the average Westerner has way too many omega-6 fatty acids in their bodies with a decided lack of omega-3's. ◆ *We need a balance of fats in our diets, not just one kind.*

Cold water fish are the best sources for EPA (and DHA, or docosochexaenoic acid): salmon, sardines, albacore, cod, butterfish, mackerel, herring, and shrimp and are the preferred source for fish oils for diabetics whose blood sugar can be elevated by fish oil supplements. Free range eggs are a good source as well. There are no vegetable sources for EPA or DHA, but flax oil, walnuts, and dark green leafy vegetables supply alpha-linolenic acid, an omega-3 fatty acid that most people can convert into EPA and DHA as needed. You should know, however, that several things can interfere with this process, including smoking, alcohol, and certain drugs, and that people from Northern European or Inuit descent usually lack the desaturating enzymes needed to create EPA or DHA in the body. For these people, then, fish and eggs are a required part of the diet (Fallon and Enig, "Tripping Lightly Down…, 3").

GLA is usually obtained in supplemental evening primrose oil, but borage and black currant oils contain higher amounts.

Fish oils have received a lot of attention recently for their proven effect in treating schizophrenia, as well as heart disease and other ailments including arthritis, asthma, lupus, and gout. Both EPA and GLA can help with menstrual irregularities and multiple sclerosis.

Food is probably your best source for EPA and DHA, but GLA is rarely found, except in human breast milk. Borage and black currant oil supplements are available in most health food stores. Cod liver oil is also readily available over the counter and is an excellent source of EPA and DHA, as well as vitamins A and D.

CARNITINE

L-carnitine is a B vitamin-like substance classified as an amino acid. L-carnitine transports fatty acids into muscular mitochondria where they are burned as energy. ◆ *L-carnitine deficiency results, then, in poor energy production.* Since the heart excels at using saturated fatty acids (especially stearic acid, found in lamb and beef fat) for energy, l-carnitine helps to keep the heart at optimal performance. Since all the body's vital organs (liver, kidney, etc.) like using fat for energy, l-carnitine helps those organs as well, preventing fatty build-up especially in the liver.

L-carnitine has been shown to help resolve and treat heart disease. According to Liberman and Bruning, the nutrient normalizes heartbeat, reduces heart cell death in heart attack victims, and reduces deaths from myocarditis. Like niacin and EPA, l-carnitine also lowers blood triglyceride levels.

Although the body can manufacture l-carnitine (only if it has enough lysine, vitamin's C, B3, B6, and the mineral iron), this nutrient is only found in animal protein, especially lamb. Vegans, then, are at risk for a deficiency.

Although no serious side effects have been observed from high doses (2-3 grams/day) of l-carnitine, it is best to seek the help of a naturopath or nutritionist in determining the optimal level for you.

CONCLUSION

It should be obvious that a varied diet of whole, unprocessed foods is one's best insurance against heart disease. Such a diet will provide all of the nutrients necessary for a strong heart and body. Remember that including refined sugars, margarine, and vegetable oils in your diet is a prescription for disease and to avoid them whenever possible. Remember as well that heart disease is a condition with many causes. If problems arise, however, one can rely on Nature's medicines to heal one's heart, mind, and body.

KEYS POINTS TO REMEMBER

♦ *A naturopath can be a very useful complement to conventional allopathic therapy.*

♦ *Herbalists through the ages have long known of several plants that act favorably on the heart muscle and circulatory system.*

♦ *Niacin is a vasodilator and increases peripheral circulation.*

♦ *CoQ10 is not only appropriate for existing cardiovascular disorders, but also as a heart disease preventive as well.*

♦ *We need a balance of fats in our diets, not just one kind.*

♦ *L-carnitine deficiency results, then, in poor energy production.*

Bibliography

Abrams,Jr., H. Leon
"Sugar—A Cultural Complex and Its Impact on Modern Society," *Jnl of Appl Nutr*, 27:2, Fall 1975.
"Vegetarianism: An Anthropological/Nutritional Evaluation," *Jnl of Appl Nutr*, 32:2, 1980.
"The Preference for Animal Protein and Fat: A Cross-Cultural Survey," in *Food and Evolution, Toward a Theory of Human Food Habits*, Marvin Harris and Eric Ross, eds., (Temple University Press; PA), 1987.
"Beware of Coffee, Tea, and Cola Beverages if You Value Your Health," *Consumer's Research*, May 1977.

Atkins, R.
Dr. Atkins' New Diet Revolution, (M. Evans and Co.; NY), 1992.

Balch, James and Balch, Phyllis
Prescription for Nutritional Healing (Avery Publishing; NY), 1995.

Brzosko, WJ & Ianowski, A.
"Padma 28 and Chronic Hepatitis B Infection." *Swiss Jnl of Holistic Medicine* 1992;4 (Suppl. 1):13-14.

Burkitt, D.P.
Cancer 28:3, 1971.

Byrnes, Stephen
"Facing the Facts About Saturated Fat," *Jnl of Amer Natur Med Assoc*, Winter 1998.

Capper, Arthur
The Searchlight Recipe Book, 25th ed. (Capper Publications; KS), 1955.

Castelli, William
"Concerning the Possibility of a Nut...," *Arch of Inter Med*, 152(7): 1371-1372, July 1992.

Cha, Y. & Sachan, S.
Jnl Amer Coll Nutr, 13(4): 338-343, August 1994.

Cranton, E.M., & Frackelton, J.
"Free Radical Pathology in Age-Associated Diseases," *Jnl of Hol Med*, Spring/Summer 1984.

Cristakis, G.
"Effect of the Anti-Coronary Club Program on Coronary heart Disease Risk-Factor Status," *Jnl of Amer Med Assoc*, 198 (6), Nov. 7, 1966.

DeBakey, Michael, et al.
"Serum Cholesterol Values in Patients Treated Surgically for Atherosclerosis," *Jnl of Amer Med Assoc*, 189 (9): 655-659, 1964.

DeFronzo & Ferrannini
Diabetes Care, 4(3): 173-194, 1991.

Douglass, William Campbell
The Milk Book. (Second Opionion; GA.), 1994.

Bibliography

Enig, Mary
"Fat Facts," *The PPNF Journal,* Winter 1998.

"Modification of Membrane Lipid Composition and Mixed-Function Oxidases in Mouse Liver Microsomes by Dietary Trans Fatty Acids," Doctoral Dissertation for the University of Maryland, 1984.

"Dietary Fat and Cancer Trends—A Critique," *Federation Proceedings,* July 1978.

"Fatty Acid Composition of the Fat in Selected Food Items...," *Jnl of Amer Oil Chem Soc,* 60(10): 1983.

Know Your Fats (Bethesda Press; 2000).

Fallon, Sally
"Nasty, Brutish, and Short?" *The Ecologist,* (London, England), 29:1, Jan/Feb 1999

Fallon, Sally, & Enig, Mary
"Merrie Olde England," *The PPNF Journal,* 21:4, Winter 1997.

"Americans: Then and Now," *The PPNF Journal,* 20:4, Winter 1996.

"Tripping Lightly Down the Prostaglandin Pathways," *The PPNF Journal,* 20:3, Fall 1996.

"The Oiling of America," *Nexus Magazine,* (Australia), Dec/Jan 1998, Feb/March 1999.

"Diet and Heart Disease: Not What You Think," *Consumers Research,* July 1996.

"Soy Products for Dairy Products? Not So Fast," *Health Freedom News,* June 1995

Fallon, Enig, & Connoly
Nourishing Traditions, (ProMotion Publishing; CA), 1995.

Felton, C.V., et al.
"Dietary Polyunsaturated Fatty Acids and Composition of Human Aortic Plaques," *Lancet,* 344:1195, 1994.

Fitzpatrick, Mike
"Soy Isoflavones: Panacea or Poison?" *The PPNF Journal,* 22:3, Fall 1998.

Gaby, A.
"Does Estrogen Replacement Therapy Prevent Heart Disease?" *Townsend Letter for Doctors & Patients,* August/September 2000, 108-109.

Garg, M. L., et al.
The FASEB Journal, 2(4), A852, 1988.

Garrison, Jr., & Somer, Elizabeth
The Nutrition Desk Reference, 3rd ed. (Keats Publishing; CT.), 1995.

Gazella, Kathryn
"Homocysteine," *Nature's Impact,* 1998.

"Heart Disease: The Possible Dairy-Sugar Connection," *Nature's Impact,* Feb/March 1999.

Gittleman, Ann Louise, et al.
Your Body Knows Best. (Pocket Books; NY), 1997.

Golomb, B. A.
"Cholesterol and Violence: Is There a Connection?" *Annals of Intern Med,* 128, 478-487, 1998.

Gurr, Michael
"A Fresh Look at Dietary Recommendations," *Inform* (7) 4: 432-435, April 1996.

Hassig, A.; Liang, W.; and Stampflik, K.
"Thoughts on the Pathogenesis and Prevention of AIDS." *Swiss Jnl of Holistic Medicine*, July 1995. Posted on www.virusmyth.com.

Hitchcock & Gracey
"Diet and Serum Cholesterol," *Arch of Dis of Chilhd*, 52:790, 1977.

Hoffer, Abram, & Walker, Morton
Putting It All Together: The New Orthmolecular Nutrition. (Keats Publushing; CT), 1996.

Jnl of Amer Med Assoc
248(12):1465, September 24, 1982.

251:359, 1984.

Jackson & Teague
The Handbook of Alternatives to Chemical Medicine, (Lawton and Teague; CA), 1985.

Jennings, Isobel
Vitamins in Endocrine Metabolism. (Charles Thomas; London), 1970.

Kabara, J.
The Pharmacological Effects of Lipids, (AOCS; IL), 1978.

Keys, Ancel
"Diet and Development of Coronary Heart Disease," *Jnl of Chron Dis.*, October 1956.

Kronmal, R.
Jnl of Amer Med Assoc, 248(12): 1465.

Kummerow, Frederick
"Effects of Isomeric Fats on Animal Tissue, Lipid Classes and Atherosclerosis," in *Geometrical and Positional Fatty Acid Isomers*, Emken and Dutton, eds, Americal Oil Chemists Society, 1979.

Kummerow & Navidi
"Nutritional Value of Egg Beaters Compared with Farm Fresh Eggs," *Pediatrics*, 53:565-566, 1974.

Lancet
350:11, 1997.

Langer, Stephen and Scheer, J.
Solved: The Riddle of Illness. (Keats Publishing; CT), 1995.

Lieberman, Shari & Bruning, Nancy
The Real Vitamin and Mineral Book. (Avery Publishing; NY), 1997..

Lindberg, G., et al.
"Low Serum Cholesterol Concentration and Short Term Mortality from Injuries in Men and Women." *Brit Med Jnl*, 305:277-279, 1992.

Mann, George, et al.
"Atherosclerosis in the Masai, *Amer Jnl Epidemiol*, 95:6-37, 1972.

Coronary Heart Disease: The Dietary Sense and Nonsense, (Veritas Society, London), 1993.

"Metabolic Consequences of Dietary Trans Fatty Acids," *Lancet* 343: 1268-1271, 1994.

McGill, H.C., et al.
"General Findings of the International Atherosclerosis Project," *Lab Invest*, 18(5): 498, 1968.

Mead, J.F., et al.
Lipids: Chemistry, Biochemistry, and Nutrition, (Plenum Press; NY), 1986.

Mudd, Chris
Cholesterol and Your Health. (American Lite Co.; OK), 1990.

Muldoon, M.F., Manuck, S.B.; Matthews, K.A.
"Lowering Cholesterol Concentrations and Mortality: A Quantitative Review of Primary Prevention Trials." *Brit Med Jnl* 301:309-314, 1990.

Nanji, A. A., et al
Gastroenterology, 109(2): 547-554, August 1995.

New Engl Jnl of Med.
98:317-323, 1978.

Oliart Ros, R. M., et al.
"Meeting Abstracts," *AOCS Proceedings,* May 199

Olson, R. E.
"Evolution of Ideas About the Nutritonal Value of Dietary Fat," *Jnl of Nutr,* 128:421S-425S, 1998.

Ornish, Dean
Stress, Diet, and Your Heart. (Holt, Rinehart and Winston; NY), 1982.

Page, M. & Abrams, H.L.
Your Body is Your Best Doctor, (Keats Publishing; CT), 1974.

Pauling, Linus
How to Live Longer and Feel Better. (Avon Books; NY), 1985.

Porter, et al.
Am. Jnl of Clin Nutr, 30:490, 1960.

Price, Weston
Nutrition & Physical Degeneration. (Keats Publishing; CT.), 1989.

Notes from Yesteryear: "Are the Activators Revealing the Nature of Life in Health and Disease Including Dental Disease?" Reprinted in Wise Traditions in Food, Farming, and the Healing Arts, Summer 2000, 19-24.

Price-Pottenger Nutrition Foundation
"Health Vectors," *The PPNF Journal.* (Price-Pottenger Nutrition Foundation; CA), 21:2, Summer 1997.

Ravnskov, Uffe
The Cholesterol Myths (New Trends Publishing, Washington, D.C.), 2000.

Reaven, G.
Diabetes, 37: 1595-1607, 1988.

Reiser, Raymond
"The Three Weak Links in the Diet-Heart Disease Connection," *Nutrition Today,* 14:22-28, 1979.

Rizek, R.L., et al.
"Fat in Today's Food Supply—Level of Use and Sources," *Jnl Amer Oil Chem Soc,* 51:244, 1974.

Rona, Zoltan
"Unnecessary Medical Tests," *Health Naturally,* Dec/Jan 1999.

Rose, G., et al.

Lancet, 1983, 1:1062-1065.

Rowland, David

The Nutritional Bypass. (Health Naturally Publications; Canada), 1995.

"Vegetarian or Carnivore?" *Health Naturally*, Aug/Sep 1999.

Slater, et al.

Nutr Report Inter, 14:249, 1975.

Smith, Russel & Pinckney, E.

Diet, Blood Cholesterol, and Coronary Heart Disease: A Critical Review of the Literature. (Vector Enterprises; CA), 1991.

The Cholesterol Conspiracy (Warren H. Green, Inc; MO), 1991.

Spencer, Herta & Kramer, Lois

"Factors Contributing to Osteoporosis," *Jnl of Nutr*, 116:316-319, 1986.

"Further Studies of the Effect of a High Protein Diet as Meat on Calcium Metabolism," *Amer Jnl Clin Nutr*, June 924-929, 1983.

Stamler, Jeremiah

Your Heart Has Nine Lives. (American Heart Association), 1966.

Stefansson, V.

The Fat of the Land, (MacMillan Publishing; NY), 1956.

Sullivan, Krispin

"The Miracle of Vitamin D." Wise Traditions in Food, Farming, and the Healing Arts, Fall 2000, 52-61.

Tasker, F.

"A Churning Controversy," *The Washington Post*, June 2, 1997.

Various

The Baptists Ladies' Cookbook, (Monmouth; IL), 1895.

The Boston Cooking School Cookbook, (Boston, MA), 1896.

The Jewish Housewives' Cookbook (London; Eng), 1847.

Watkins, B., et al.

"Importance of Vitamin E in Bone Formation and in Chondrocyte Function," *AOCS Proceedings*, 1996.

Watkins & Seifert

"Food Lipids and Bone Health," in *Food Lipids and Health*, McDonald and Min, eds., (Marcel Dekker, Inc; NY).

Williams, Roger

Nutrition Against Disease, (Bantam Books; NY), 1973.

Wolk, et al.

Arch of Intern Med, 158:41, 1998.

Yudkin, John

Pure, White, and Deadly. (Davis Poynter; London), 1972.

"Sugar Consumption and Myocardial Infarction," *Lancet* 1:296-297, 1971.

Bibliography

"Sucrose and Heart Disease," *Lancet* 14:16-20, 1969.

"Sugar Intake and Myocardial Infarction," *Am Jnl Clin Nutr,* 20: 503, 1967.

"Dietary Fat and Dietary Sugar in Relation to Ishemic Heart Disease and Diabetes," *Lancet,* 2:4, 1964.

Zavoroni, I., et al.
New Eng Jnl of Med, 320:702-706, 1989.

Index

Resources

CANADA:

The International Organisation of Nutritional Consultants (IONC), 1201 Division St., Kingston, Ontario K7K 6X4. Phone: (613) 382-8161. Email: ncoc@king.igs.net. The INOC can provide referrals to registered nutritionists throughout Canada and some foreign countries. The IONC confers the designation RNCP, registered nutritional consulting practitioner.

AMERICA:

The American Naturopathic Medical Association, PO Box 96273, Las Vegas, NV. 89193. Phone: (702) 897-7053. Web: www.anmaamerica.com. The ANMA is the largest and oldest naturopathic professional organization in the United States and can provide referrals to certified naturopaths and naturopathic physicians throughout the USA and foreign countries.

The Weston A. Price Foundation, PMB Box 106-380, 4200 Wisconsin Ave, NW, Washington, D.C., 20016. Web: www.westonaprice.org. The website has numerous articles and technical papers on nutrition available for downloading.

COOKBOOKS:

Nourishing Traditions by Sally Fallon and Mary Enig. Available from New Trends Publishing, 1-877-707-1776.

WEBSITES:

www.powerhealth.net is the author's personal website. Go here for info on my FREE e-zine, counseling services, nutritional and healthy living guides, and degree programs in Nutrition & Natural Therapies.

www.soyonlineservice.co.nz has numerous abstracts and summaries on soybeans, soy isoflavones, and current soy studies.

www.mercola.com offers a free, weekly health newsletter delivered to your personal Email. You can subscribe through the site. The site also contains numerous articles on soybeans, root canals, and more.

www.azomite.com is the website for Azomite Mineral Products. A superb trace mineral supplement. You can also call 1-877-296-6483.

AUTHOR:

My email is **drbyrnes@hotmail.com**. Contact me with any questions regarding the Arterial Cleansing Formula, or my many publications on AIDS, homeopathy, herbal medicine, health myths, vegetarianism, nutrition, and children's health.